For Layla & H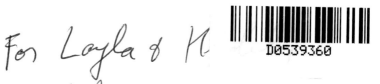
Feb. 2006
Love from
Ian

Our friends &

partners ——

Gynaecological Urology for the MRCOG and Beyond

Published titles in this series

Antenatal Disorders for the MRCOG and Beyond *by Andrew Thomson and Ian Greer*

Fetal Medicine for the MRCOG and Beyond *by Alan Cameron, Lena Macara, Janet Brennand and Peter Milton*

Gynaecological and Obstetric Pathology for the MRCOG *by Harold Fox and C. Hilary Buckley, with a chapter on Cervical Cytology by Dulcie V. Coleman*

Gynaecological Oncology for the MRCOG and Beyond *edited by David Luesley and Nigel Acheson*

Intrapartum Care for the MRCOG and Beyond *by Thomas F. Baskett and Sabaratnam Arulkumaran, with a chapter on Neonatal Resuscitation by John McIntyre and a chapter on Perinatal Loss by Carolyn Basak*

Management of Infertility for the MRCOG and Beyond *by Allan A. Templeton et al.*

Menopause for the MRCOG and Beyond *by Margaret Rees*

Medical Genetics for the MRCOG and Beyond *by Michael Connor*

Menstrual Problems for the MRCOG *by Mary Ann Lumsden, Jane Norman and Hilary Critchley*

Neonatology for the MRCOG *by Peter Dear and Simon Newell*

Reproductive Endocrinology for the MRCOG and Beyond *edited by Adam Balen*

The MRCOG: A Guide to the Examination *by Ian Johnson et al.*

Forthcoming titles in the series

Early Pregnancy Issues

Haemorrhage and Thrombosis

Molecular Medicine

Psychological Disorders in Obstetrics and Gynaecology

Gynaecological Urology for the MRCOG and Beyond

Simon Jackson MA MD MRCOG
Consultant Gynaecologist, Oxford Radcliffe Hospitals NHS
Trust, Women's Centre, John Radcliffe Hospital,
Headington, Oxford OX3 9DU, UK

Meghana Pandit MRCOG
Specialist Registrar, Oxford Radcliffe Hospitals NHS Trust,
Women's Centre, John Radcliffe Hospital, Headington,
Oxford OX3 9DU, UK

Alexandra Blackwell MRCOG
Specialist Registrar, Oxford Radcliffe Hospitals NHS Trust,
Women's Centre, John Radcliffe Hospital, Headington,
Oxford OX3 9DU, UK

RCOG Press

Published by the **RCOG Press** at the Royal College of Obstetricians and Gynaecologists, 27 Sussex Place, Regent's Park, London NW1 4RG

www.rcog.org.uk

Registered charity no. 213280

First published 2005

ISBN 1-900364-88-3

RCOG Editor: Elisabeth Rees Evans
Design/typesetting by Karl Harrington, FiSH Books, London
Index by Liza Furnival, Medical Indexing Ltd

Printed by Latimer Trend & Co. Ltd, Estover Road, Plymouth PL6 7PL, UK

Cover illustration: Vaginal cones

Acknowledgements
Thanks to Paul Moran and Jonathan Duckitt, who kindly helped provide illustrations for the book.

Contents

Abbreviations

CFU	colony-forming unit
CT	computed tomography
IVU	intravenous urography
MRI	magnetic resonance imaging
MUCP	maximum urethral closure pressure
pabd	intra-abdominal pressure
pdet	detrusor pressure
pura	urethral closure pressure
pres	intravesical pressure
TVT	tension free vaginal tape

Introduction

While the upper renal tract remains the sole preserve of the urologist, gynaecologists in addition to urologists have traditionally been involved in the assessment and treatment of female lower urinary tract symptoms. There are sound reasons for this; childbirth is a major aetiological factor, and women often present with a combination of menstrual, genital, urinary and colorectal symptoms which require a holistic approach. It is for this reason that the subspecialty of urogynaecology has arisen. Clinicians who deal with such women require a thorough understanding of the assessment and treatment of bladder filling and storage disorders, genitourinary prolapse and colorectal disorders and need to work closely with allied professions. This text aims to introduce those aspects of urology that clinicians are likely to encounter in their capacity as general obstetricians and gynaecologists. References are provided to guide the interested clinician who wishes to comprehensively review a particular subject.

1 Urinary incontinence: a common and debilitating condition

The gynaecologist with an interest in female urology will see women with a range of symptoms, including urinary frequency, both daytime and nocturnal, urgency, incomplete bladder emptying, poor urinary stream, recurrent 'cystitis' and bladder pain. Many of these symptoms coexist but the majority of referrals will include the symptom of urinary incontinence. Unlike many of the other above symptoms, the prevalence of this condition has been well documented; furthermore, some work has been done assessing the impact of urinary incontinence on lifestyle or 'quality of life'.

Prevalence

Urinary incontinence is 'the complaint of any involuntary leakage of urine'.[1] Estimates of prevalence vary considerably according to the different populations studied and the differing definitions of urinary incontinence used. Urinary incontinence should be further described by specifying factors such as frequency and severity of incontinent episodes. Feneley et al.,[2] using a definition of incontinence as two or more episodes of leakage within the previous month, reported a prevalence of 8% among females aged 5 years and over in the community while Harrison and Memel[3] reported a prevalence of 53% among a similar population of women aged 20 and above; whether, in this latter study, there was any cut-off frequency below which a diagnosis of incontinence was not made was not specified. Swithinbank et al.[4] reported an even higher rate among community dwelling women aged 18 years and above, 69% having had some degree of incontinence within the previous month. Impact from the condition should be assessed and this study was one of the few to include a measure of symptom 'bother'; 30% of the women indicated they had incontinence that had a social or hygienic impact.

Not everyone with incontinence is sufficiently bothered by their symptom to want help; it has been estimated that approximately half of all sufferers, equating to one in ten women and one in 30 men aged over 35 years, would welcome some form of treatment.[5] However, there is reluctance to seek help: only about one-third of regularly incontinent women discuss their problem with a nurse or general practitioner. Twenty percent of women referred to a urodynamic clinic have delayed seeking their general practitioner's advice for more than five years after their symptoms have become troublesome,[6] although this may have improved over the past decade as a consequence of patient education. Reasons cited for the reluctance to seek help include low expectations of treatment, thinking incontinence is a usual woman's complaint or not a serious problem, and being too embarrassed. The medical profession may do little to dispel these misconceptions: although the majority of women who discuss their condition with their GP feel that they are treated sympathetically, 30% of women who discuss their problems with a healthcare professional receive no assessment and about 80% are not examined.[7]

Quality of life

Evaluation of urinary incontinence has, until now, relied upon symptom assessment by a physician and objective diagnostic tests – usually pad testing or urodynamics. However, many factors other than the severity of urinary leakage affect the perception of incontinence as a significant health problem. These include age, culture, social class, interpersonal relationships, social support, underlying aetiology, duration of symptoms and other current illnesses. Some method of measuring the effect incontinence has on an individual is desirable.

MEASURING 'QUALITY OF LIFE'

While the ethos of quality of life was clearly embodied in the constitution of the World Health Organization as early as 1947, when health was defined as 'a state of physical, social and mental wellbeing', measuring such an ambiguous, subjective and multidimensional concept is problematic. Essentially there are two approaches to measuring quality of life. First, a general profile of health status can be obtained by measuring physical, psychological and social health. The SF-36 Health Status Questionnaire is an example of such an approach and is called a generic instrument.[8] Generic instruments are designed to measure functioning and wellbeing in a broad range of populations, are not specific to any particular condition and therefore allow comparisons between different clinical conditions and populations. However, they do not determine what impact a given condition is having on an individual's lifestyle.

Women with urinary incontinence are often otherwise in good health and generic health scores therefore tend to be low.

Alternatively, disease-specific measures can be used. These are developed to target a specific condition or group of conditions and allow more in-depth assessment of specific symptoms and concerns pertinent to that particular population. Instruments developed to assess female incontinence and other related lower urinary tract symptoms include the Kings Health Questionnaire[9] and the Bristol Female Lower Urinary Tract Symptoms Questionnaire.[10,11]

IMPACT OF URINARY INCONTINENCE ON QUALITY OF LIFE

Continent women have been reported to have higher levels of emotional wellbeing, with wellbeing decreasing in proportion to the severity of incontinence; affected individuals score highly for emotional disturbance and social isolation.[12] Incontinence secondary to detrusor overactivity has greater impact than that due to sphincter weakness, with activities involving unfamiliar places with unknown toilet availability having the greatest impact. For example, shopping where toilet availability is uncertain and coach travel with no toilet facilities would impact highly. The reasons why urge incontinence appears to be more distressing than stress incontinence may include associated urinary urgency, frequency and nocturia, more severe leakage with the bladder frequently voiding completely off an unstable detrusor contraction, and the inability to predict incontinent episodes and hence avoid precipitating factors. As a result, many aspects of normal lifestyle are avoided and a new way of life develops that is organised around toilet location and avoiding potentially embarrassing situations. Younger women experience greatest impact, with sleep and rest, emotional behaviour, mobility, social interaction and recreational activities being particularly affected.[6]

Conclusion

Prevalence studies have differed markedly in the populations studied and the methods used. As a consequence, published figures for urinary incontinence vary considerably. However, whichever estimates are used, urinary incontinence is undoubtedly common in apparently healthy women and, although the science of measuring quality of life is still in its infancy, incontinence undoubtedly causes considerable distress. There is much that can be done to cure or alleviate both incontinence and other lower urinary tract symptoms and these measures will be addressed in the subsequent chapters.

References

1. Abrams P, Cardozo L, Fall M, Griffiths D, Rosier P, Ulmsten U, *et al*. The standardisation or terminology of lower urinary tract function: report from the Standardisation Subcommittee of the International Continence Society. *Neurourol Urodyn* 2002;21:167–78.
2. Feneley RC, Shepherd AM, Powell PH, Blannin J. Urinary incontinence: prevalence and needs. *Br J Urol* 1979;51:493–6.
3. Harrison GL, Memel DS. Urinary incontinence in women: its prevalence and its management in a health promotion clinic. *Br J Gen Pract* 1994;44:149–52.
4. Swithinbank LV, Donovan JL, du Heaume JC, Rogers CA, James MC, Yang Q, *et al*. Urinary symptoms and incontinence in women: relationships between occurrence, age and perceived impact. *Br J Gen Pract* 1999;49:897–900.
5. O'Brien J, Austin M, Sethi P, O'Boyle P. Urinary incontinence: prevalence, need for treatment and effectiveness of intervention by nurse. *BMJ* 1991;303:1308–12.
6. Norton PA, MacDonald LD, Sedgwick PM, Stanton SL. Distress and delay associated with urinary incontinence, frequency and urgency in women. *BMJ* 1988;297:1187–9.
7. Brocklehurst JC. Urinary incontinence in the community: analysis of a MORI poll. *BMJ* 1993;306:832–4.
8. Brazier JE, Harper R, Jones NMB, *et al*. Validating the SF-36 health survey questionnaire: a new outcome measure for primary care. *BMJ* 1992;305:160–64.
9. Kelleher CJ, Cardozo LD, Toozs-Hobson PM. Quality of life and urinary incontinence. *Curr Opin Obstet Gynecol* 1995;7:404–8.
10. Jackson S, Donovan J, Brookes S, Eckford S, Swithinbank L, Abrams P. The Bristol Female Lower Urinary Tract Symptoms questionnaire: development and psychometric testing. *Br J Urol* 1996;77:805–12.
11. Brookes St, Donovan JL, Wright M, Jackson S, Abrams P. A scored form of the Bristol Female Lower Urinary Tract Stmptoms Questionnaire: data from a randomised control trial of surgery for women with stress incontinence. Am J Obstet Gynecol 2004;191:73–82.
12. Grimby A, Milsom I, Molander U, Wiklund I, Ekelund P. The influence of urinary incontinence on the QoL of elderly women. *Age Ageing* 1993;22:82–9.

2   Applied anatomy

A detailed description of formal anatomy is beyond the scope of this text and of limited interest to the general clinician. There are, however, certain aspects of anatomy that are of particular clinical relevance and should be familiar to everyone working within this field.

Normal lower urinary tract function depends, during the filling phase of the cycle, upon adequate bladder capacity and a competent urethral sphincter. The voiding phase is dependent upon detrusor contractility and coordinated urethral relaxation.

The bladder

The bladder has to be highly compliant to enable urine storage without significant rises in intravesical pressure. The extracellular matrix of elastin, collagen and intercellular ground substance determines much of the bladder's viscoelastic properties. In addition, the bladder wall consists of smooth muscle bundles. As the detrusor muscle has an outer longitudinal layer, and inner oblique and circular layers, it can be divided into the more distensible dome and a thicker, less distensible base. The mucosal lining is transitional and the urinary trigone has its apices at the ureteric orifices and the internal urinary meatus. The ureters pass obliquely through the muscle wall of the bladder; this prevents vesico-ureteric reflux of urine. The innervation of the bladder is predominantly autonomic, the parasympathetics stimulating detrusor contractility while the sympathetics maintain urethral sphincter tone.

The urethra

The urethra is a complex muscular tube, 3–4 cm long. The urethral wall comprises the outer striated urogenital muscle also referred to as the rhabdosphincter or the striated sphincter. This striated muscle surrounds circular and longitudinal smooth muscle fibres. Additional extrinsic occlusion is provided by striated periurethral muscle and the levator ani muscles; this is thought to account for urethral closure at times of physical effort. There is sympathetic innervation of the urethral sphincter and stimulation increases urethral closure pressure.

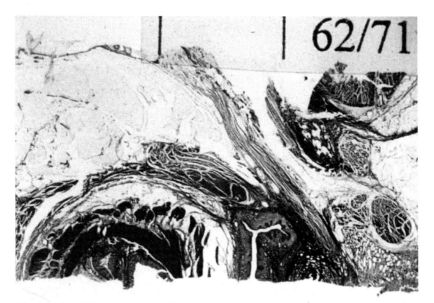

Figure 2.1 Histological section through urethra showing mucosa, submucosa and smooth muscle

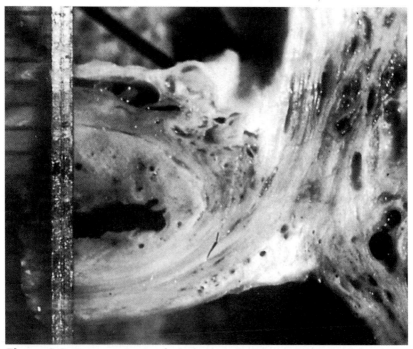

Figure 2.2 Gross anatomy of urethral section shown in Figure 2.1

Lying between the urethral mucosa and the smooth muscle is the submucosa with its rich vascular supply (Figures 2.1 and 2.2). A watertight seal is derived from close apposition of the rugose surfaces of the urothelium; this is striated squamous in its distal third and transitional in the proximal part. The urothelium is hormone sensitive, oestrogen receptors being present.[1]

The continence mechanism

Continence depends upon intrinsic urethral sphincter tone, providing urethral closure pressure and pelvic floor support. A number of theories have been proposed to explain female continence.

INTRINSIC URETHRAL SPHINCTER FUNCTION

The urethral striated and smooth muscle, in combination with the submucosal urethral vascular plexus, all contribute to providing occlusive pressure and maintaining mucosal apposition. Urethral closure pressure decreases with age. This may be owing to muscle atrophy, reduced nerve fasicles in the striated sphincter,[2] reducing submucosal blood flow or trophic changes to the urothelium. Oestrogen may prevent some of these changes although this is controversial.

INTRA-ABDOMINAL PRESSURE TRANSMISSION

The proximal urethra is positioned above the pelvic floor and is thus intra-abdominal. Increases in intra-abdominal pressure will be transmitted equally to the bladder and the proximal urethra, resulting in a simultaneous increase in intravesical and urethral pressure, thus preventing urinary leakage (Figures 2.3 and 2.4). While this may undoubtedly be one factor contributing to the maintenance of continence, the theory is excessively simplistic. Its role as the pre-dominant mechanism can be discredited because not all women with bladder neck hypermobility and poor anterior vaginal wall support are incontinent.

VAGINAL HAMMOCK

The vagina has been compared to a hammock, supporting the urethra, transmitting increases in intra-abdominal pressure and promoting urethral closure. This is dependent upon the vagina being attached to the pelvic sidewall. Studies based on cadaveric dissection[3] have shown that the vagina has two lateral attachments: a fascial attachment to the

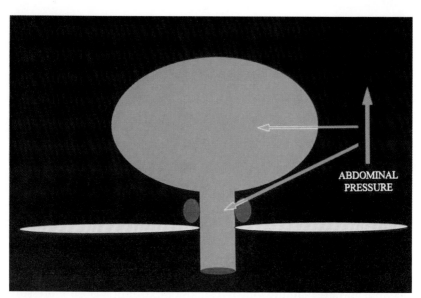

Figure 2.3 If the proximal urethra is positioned above the pelvic floor, increases in intra-abdominal pressure will be transmitted equally to the bladder and the proximal urethra, thus preventing urinary leakage

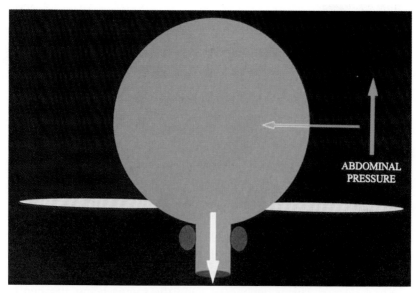

Figure 2.4 If the proximal urethra prolapses beyond the pelvic floor, the pressure transmission to the proximal urethra does not occur, thus predisposing to incontinence

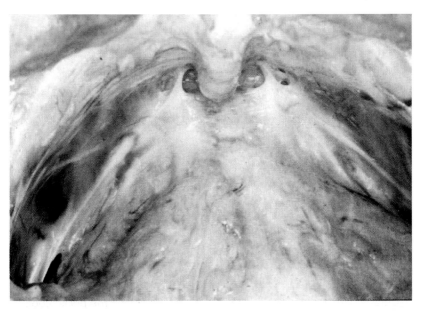

Figure 2.5 Normal fascia attachments between the vagina and the arcus tendineus fascia pelvis; the vagina thus provides support for the bladder

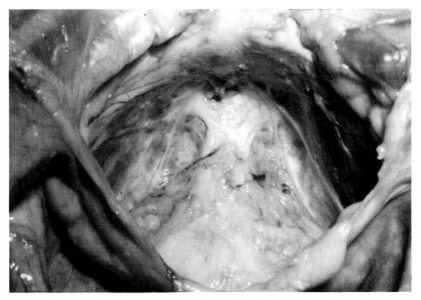

Figure 2.6 The fascia attachments have failed, the vagina is no longer attached to the arcus tendineus and the bladder is poorly supported, thus predisposing to incontinence

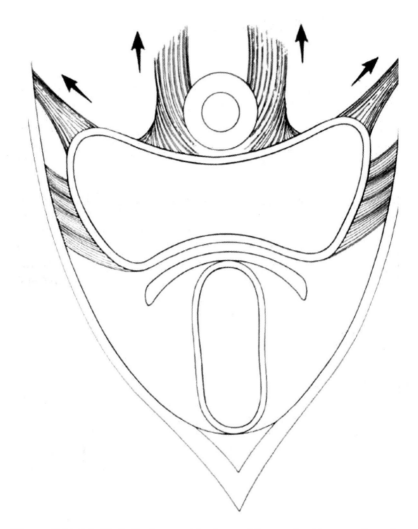

Figure 2.7 It is likely that a combination of the vaginal hammock and urethral support via the pubo-urethral ligament is important for maintaining continence

arcus tendineus fascia pelvis and a muscular attachment to the medial border of the levator ani (Figures 2.5 and 2.6). When there is an increase in abdominal pressure, the urethra is compressed against the hammock created by the endopelvic fascia and the anterior vaginal wall. The stability of this fascial layer determines the effectiveness of the urethral closure mechanism against rising abdominal pressure (Figure 2.7).

Aspects of clinical relevance

BLADDER

- Squamous metaplasia of the trigone is a common finding at cystoscopy and is a variant of normal (Figure 2.8).

- Bladder compliance is reduced by interstitial cystitis (Figure 2.9). Bladder capacities are reduced and hypersensitivity is present. The diagnosis is made by cystoscopy and bladder biopsy. Mast cells are typically seen.

- Detrusor overactivity secondary to neurological pathology (neurogenic detrusor overactivity) can cause hypertrophy of the bladder wall. The reduced compliance and high intravesical pressures generated place the upper renal tracts at risk and such women should be assessed for evidence of ureteric reflux and renal cortical scarring; if present cystoplasty is required to reduce intravesical pressures and preserve the renal function.

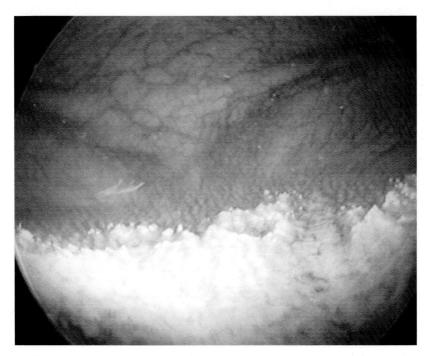

Figure 2.8 Squamous metaplasia of the trigone

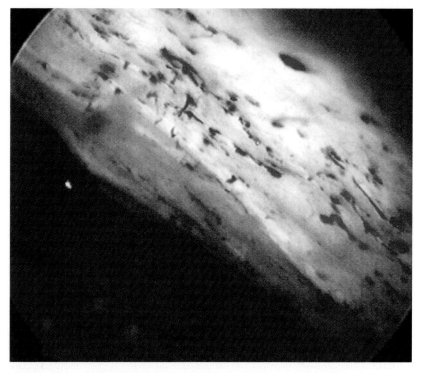

Figure 2.9 Typical features of interstitial cystitis on cystoscopy. The mucosa has split during bladder distension and areas of haemorrhage can be seen

- Neurological pathology such as multiple sclerosis will sometimes present initially with lower urinary tract symptoms and, although most detrusor overactivity is idiopathic, if there are other factors such as loss of coordination between the detrusor and urethra during voiding (detrusor–sphincter dyssynergia) or other associated neurological symptoms, further investigation with magnetic resonance imaging (MRI) of the lumbar and sacral cord is warranted.

- The bladder when full becomes intra-abdominal; drainage is therefore required before performing a low abdominal incision. If major bladder injury is sustained at the time of surgery it is vital that the trigone is visualised, the ureters are identified and ureteric injury is excluded; if there is doubt ureteric stenting and retrograde radiography will be required.

- Should bladder rupture or urinary extravasation occur at the time of endoscopic surgery a cystogram will be required to determine whether the urinary leakage is extra- or intraperitoneal. Intraperitoneal rupture requires a laparotomy while extraperitoneal leakage can usually be managed with bladder drainage and antibiotics.

- Bladder overdistension may result in autonomic neuropathy. This is all too commonly seen when postpartum or postoperative retention goes unrecognised and in some cases the neuropathy results in permanent voiding dysfunction. It is therefore vital that postoperative and postpartum women receive diligent bladder care. None should be left more than six hours without the bladder being drained[4-6] and drainage should occur earlier if the woman is uncomfortable in the interim.

URETHRA

- Urethral strictures may be present if a woman has had urethral surgery or a severe urethral infection. These women, if presenting with poor stream, incomplete bladder emptying or recurrent urinary tract infections, may benefit from urethral dilatation, but in other circumstances this procedure is of doubtful benefit.

- Paraurethral cysts should be differentiated from urethral diverticula prior to surgery. Excising a diverticulum transvaginally runs the risk of creating a urethrovaginal fistula unless care is taken to prevent this by using a technique such as interposition of a Martius labial fat pad graft. Excising a paraurethral cyst carries no such risk unless the urethral wall is inadvertently incised at the time of surgery.

- When urodynamic stress incontinence is present the choice of surgery may depend upon whether the cause of the incontinence is thought to be urethral hypermobility or intrinsic sphincter deficiency.

Colposuspension restores continence by approximation of the periurethral endopelvic fascia and anterior vagina to the ileopectineal ligament thereby recreating the 'hammock'. This operation is one of our gold standards for the treatment of urinary stress incontinence but is only suitable for women who clinically have bladder neck hypermobility. Incontinence secondary to intrinsic sphincter deficiency is commonly seen in women who have had repeated vaginal surgery or in those with postmenopausal vaginal atrophy. If these women have a well-supported bladder neck they require a different surgical approach, using either urethral injection therapy or a urethral sling. It should be noted that while slings and urethral injectables are, in addition to use in women with intrinsic sphincter deficiency, also suitable for women with bladder neck hypermobility, the colposuspension is not suitable for women with a fixed bladder neck.

References

1. Blakeman PJ, Hilton P, Bulmer JN. Oestrogen and progesterone receptor expression in the female lower urinary tract, with reference to oestrogen status. *Br J Urol* 2000;86:32–8.
2. Pandit M, Delanay JOL, Ashton-Miller JA, *et al.* Quantification of intramuscular nerves within the female striated urogenital sphincter muscle. *Obstet Gynecol* 2000;95:797–800.
3. Ashton-Miller JA, Howard D, DeLancey JO. The functional anatomy of the female pelvic floor and stress incontinence control system. *Scand J Urol Nephrol Suppl* 2001;207:1–7.
4. Royal College of Obstetricians and Gynaecologists. *Clinical Standards – Advice on Planning the Service in Obstetrics and Gynaecology.* London: RCOG; 2002.
5. Department of Health. *Good Practice in Continence Services.* London: DoH; 2000.
6. Zaki M, Pandit M, Jackson S. National survey of intrapartum and postpartum bladder care: assessing the need for guidelines. *BJOG* 2004;111:874–6.

3 Lower urinary tract symptoms: initial assessment

All women with lower urinary tract symptoms must have a basic assessment which should include a clinical history and examination, urinalysis and a self-completed urinary diary. All of this can be performed within the primary care setting. Many women will be treatable at this stage. Further complex investigations can be reserved for defined subgroups; these will be described in Chapter 4.

History

It is important to prioritise the symptoms, which may include urinary incontinence, daytime frequency, nocturia, urgency, dysuria, bladder pain, haematuria, incomplete emptying, poor urinary stream and hesitancy.

CHARACTERISING INCONTINENCE

Urinary incontinence can be further characterised. Stress incontinence is the complaint of involuntary leakage on effort or exertion, or on sneezing or coughing,[1] and suggests a problem with urethral competence. Urge incontinence is the complaint of involuntary leakage accompanied by, or immediately preceded by, urgency[1] and commonly suggests there may be underlying detrusor overactivity. Other types of incontinence include nocturnal enuresis (loss of urine occurring during sleep), continuous urinary incontinence and loss of urine in specific situations, most commonly giggle incontinence and leakage with sexual intercourse.

As well as specifying the type, incontinence should be further characterised by specifying the frequency (Box 2.1) and severity of incontinent episodes. Women with detrusor overactivity often lose large volumes of urine and the loss can be completely unpredictable. Enquiring about need to change clothing and pad usage can help assess the severity of incontinence. Precipitating factors should be sought and the clinician should assess the impact of incontinence on quality of life.

Frequency implies one of the following:

- that the detrusor muscle is overactive
- that bladder capacity is reduced
- that urine production is excessive (namely polyuria, defined as measured production of more than 2.8 litres of urine in 24 hours in adults[1,2]).

Many women, however, have developed the habit of voiding frequently (for example, they may find that keeping the bladder empty protects from urinary stress incontinence) and therefore urinary frequency in isolation has little diagnostic specificity. Urgency is most frequently secondary to detrusor overactivity, although inflammatory bladder conditions such as interstitial cystitis may also present with this.

BOX 2.1. DEFINITIONS: FREQUENCY AND URGENCY

Daytime frequency:	Number of voids recorded during waking hours and includes the last void before sleep and the first void after waking and rising in the morning.[1]
Increased daytime frequency	Defined by the person's perception that he or she voids too often by day.[1]
Nocturia	Complaint that the individual has to wake at night one or more times to void.[1,2]
Urgency	Complaint of a sudden compelling desire to pass urine, which is difficult to defer.[1]

OTHER SYMPTOMS

Pain is an uncommon bladder symptom. Typically, the pain occurs with bladder filling and is relieved by emptying. This symptom suggests intravesical pathology such as interstitial cystitis or malignancy and warrants a cystoscopy.

Haematuria may be secondary to infection and this should be excluded. In the absence of infection cystoscopy, renal ultrasound and a plain abdominal radiograph are required to investigate for tumours and calculi.

Voiding symptoms, including hesitancy, slow or intermittent stream and incomplete emptying, suggest urethral obstruction, an underactive detrusor muscle or loss of coordination between detrusor contraction and urethral relaxation (detrusor–sphincter dyssynergia). This is occasionally seen with neurological disease.

Global pelvic dysfunction is commonly present and, in addition to the above, the clinician should enquire about colorectal symptoms and genitourinary prolapse (anal incontinence is still a taboo subject and may not be volunteered).

AETIOLOGICAL FACTORS

The history should aim to explore possible aetiological factors and should enquire about neurological disease, past obstetric trauma and previous gynaecological and urological surgery. A good clinical history will also enquire about disease impact. Impact on quality of life can be assessed by asking how symptoms affect aspects of daily life and social, personal and sexual relationships. A symptom that may not bother one person can have devastating impact on another; for example mild urinary stress incontinence may not trouble those with an inactive lifestyle while severely incapacitating a gymnast. A woman with frequency and urgency may cope well if her office desk is close to a toilet while debilitating a teacher who has to lecture for an hour without interruption.

Questionnaires have been developed to allow lower urinary tract symptoms, symptom severity and quality of life to be measured in a reproducible way without any bias from the interviewer.[3,4] These can be used in both clinical and research settings, enabling standardisation of symptom assessment, prioritisation of symptoms and measurement of disease severity and impact.

Physical examination

The woman with incontinence requires an abdominal examination to exclude urinary retention, a neurological assessment of the lower limbs and perineum, a bimanual examination to exclude pelvic masses and a vaginal examination. Vaginal examination should include an assessment of urethral and bladder neck descent on straining, anterior vaginal wall mobility and concurrent uterovaginal prolapse. This information is necessary before deciding on appropriate surgery, should this be necessary, and is usually performed in the left lateral position using a Sims speculum. An assessment of the pelvic floor musculature should be made, preferably by an appropriately trained physiotherapist. The assessment should include a measure of tone at rest, muscle strength with voluntary contraction and the ease with which the muscle fatigues. Validated grading systems (e.g. Oxford 1–5) allow strength to be quantified. A suitably qualified physiotherapist will know whether further treatment with a programme of pelvic floor exercises is likely to be beneficial or not. If the muscle is already strong further exercises are unlikely to prove helpful while if there is little voluntary activity pudendal nerve stimulation may be required to help initiate a contraction.

Urinary diary

Frequency of micturition and leakage episodes can be assessed using a daily diary. This is a simple and practical method of obtaining information on voiding behaviour. A frequency/volume chart records the point in time and volume of all voids over a specified period; this should include day and night and be of at least 24 hours in duration. Objective information is obtained, not only on daytime frequency and nocturia but also on normal functional bladder capacity, mean voided volume, total voided volume and diurnal distribution of micturitions. Normal values have been obtained for the asymptomatic population: women void a median of eight times in 24 hours and approximately 40% rise to void at night,[5] with a tendency for the frequency of nocturnal micturitions to increase with age.

Abnormalities seen may include frequency and nocturia. The 24-hour urine output varies immensely and may show fluid restriction (passing less than 30 ml urine per hour) or, more frequently, polyuria (passing more than 2.8 litres of urine per 24 hours). The polyuria may be global or nocturnal (where the woman passes more than one-third of her 24-hour urine output during the 8 hours of sleep) (Figure 3.1). When polyuria is present the clinician must ensure that it is not secondary to pathology such as diabetes mellitus, diabetes insipidus or hypercalcaemia. The majority will however prove to have primary polydipsia and simple advice regarding fluid restriction will be sufficient to resolve the urinary frequency.

Functional bladder capacity is another diary parameter that helps guide the clinician to underlying pathology: normal frequency and volumes may suggest sphincter weakness with healthy detrusor muscle; variable volumes with frequency are seen with detrusor overactivity; and reduced fixed volumes with frequency may indicate intravesical pathology such as interstitial cystitis.

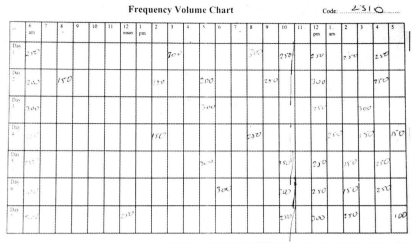

Figure 3.1 Urinary diary showing nocturnal polyuria, more than one-third of the 24-hour urine output occurring during the hours of sleep

Urinalysis and urine culture

Urinary tract infection can mimic any lower urinary tract condition causing frequency, urgency and incontinence. Urine microscopy and culture is the diagnostic gold standard, but reagent strip testing of urine for leucocyte esterase and nitrites is sensitive and provides a cheaper screening method. Bacteriological analysis is reserved for those with a positive screening test result.[6,7] In cases of haematuria urine should also be sent for cytological analysis.

Summary

The information in this chapter constitutes the initial management of a woman with lower urinary tract symptoms. Many women will need to progress no further and can be managed with simple advice and treatment. Conservative measures may include decreased caffeine consumption, reduced or increased fluid intake, pelvic floor exercises, bladder drill and anticholinergics.

References

1. Abrams P, Cardozo L, Fall M, Griffiths D, Rosier P, Ulmsten U, *et al*. The standardisation of terminology of lower urinary tract function. Report from the Standardisation Subcommittee of the International Continence Society. *Neurourol Urodyn* 2002;21:167–78.

2. Van Kerrebroeck P, Abrams P, Chaikin D, Donovan J, Fonder D, Jackson S, *et al*. The standardisation of terminology in nocturia; report from the Standardisation Committee of the International Continence Society. *Neurol Urodyn* 2002;21:179–83.

3. Kelleher CJ, Cardozo LD, Khullar V, Salvatore S. A new questionnaire to assess quality of life of urinary incontinent women. *Br J Obstet Gynaecol* 1997;104:1374–9.

4. Jackson S, Donovan J, Brookes S, Eckford S, Swithinbank L, Abrams P. The Bristol Female Lower Urinary Tract Symptoms questionnaire: development and psychometric testing. *Br J Urol* 1996;77:805–12.

5. Fitzgerald MP, Stablein U, Brubaker L. Urinary habits among asymptomatic women. *Am J Obstet Gynecol* 2002;187:1384–8.

6. Preston A, O'Donnell T, Phillips CA. Screening for urinary tract infections in a gynaecological setting: validity and cost-effectiveness of reagent strips. *Br J Biomed Sci* 1999;56:253–7.

7. Nunns D, Smith AR, Hosker G. Reagent strip testing urine for significant bacteriuria in a urodynamic clinic. *Br J Urol* 1995;76:87–9.

4 Lower urinary tract symptoms: further investigation

Some women with lower urinary tract symptoms will require more extensive investigation than that outlined in Chapter 3. Additional assessment may require any or a combination of urodynamics, cystoscopy, urinary tract imaging and perineal pad testing. It is essential that the clinical indications for these are clearly understood.

Urodynamics

A common immediate reaction of clinicians when consulted by a woman complaining of lower urinary tract symptoms is to request a urodynamic assessment. Clinicians often do not appreciate the indications for the test. They have little perception of what the study entails, they have no knowledge of its limitations and they struggle to interpret the results.

CLINICAL INDICATIONS

Complex mixed lower urinary tract symptoms

Some women present with such a complicated history that it is impossible to make any judgement as to whether they are suffering from urinary stress incontinence, detrusor overactivity or voiding dysfunction. Such women cannot be treated empirically and they should progress without delay to a urodynamic assessment so that treatment can be tailored appropriately.

Before surgery for urinary stress incontinence

Stress urinary incontinence is the most common cause of urinary leakage in women. If pelvic floor physiotherapy fails, surgery is the definitive treatment. Some clinicians claim that history alone is an adequate preoperative assessment in women presenting with pure stress incontinence symptoms.[1,2] However, even women presenting with symptoms suggesting pure stress incontinence may have detrusor overactivity as the underlying cause of their incontinence when investigated with a urodynamic assessment.[3] It has been claimed that surgery performed on the basis of symptoms alone will result in inappropriate treatment up to 27% of the time[4] and cystometry is recommended before bladder-neck surgery to confirm the presence of urodynamic stress incontinence.

There are additional equally important reasons for a preoperative urodynamic assessment. Surgery for stress incontinence can result in *de novo* detrusor overactivity[5] or exacerbate pre-existing detrusor overactivity, so an assessment of detrusor function before surgery is prudent. Women who void by straining with poor detrusor contractility, or those who empty their bladders incompletely, are at increased risk of prolonged postoperative retention. While it is essential that all women considering continence surgery are warned of the potential risk of retention, these women are at particularly high risk and it is important to teach these women to self-catheterise preoperatively. If this technique cannot be mastered, potentially obstructive bladder neck surgery is best avoided.

Women presenting with stress incontinence who have yet to try physiotherapy or who would not consider continence surgery do not require a urodynamic assessment. Cystometry in these women is unlikely to alter management: if the urodynamic study failed to confirm stress incontinence physiotherapy would still be indicated. They probably do have mild stress incontinence as the laboratory environment cannot always replicate 'real life' events, and physiotherapy is therefore entirely appropriate. Conversely, if the test did confirm urodynamic stress incontinence, it would be inappropriate to proceed directly to surgery without trying physiotherapy first.

Symptoms suggestive of detrusor overactivity

The likeliest pathology underlying urinary frequency and urgency is detrusor overactivity. This may be strongly suspected from the woman's history and frequency/volume chart. The primary treatment is bladder training and pharmacotherapy with anticholinergics. Although anticholinergic drugs may cause adverse effects, these are rapidly reversible and these drugs are essentially safe. Therefore, as inappropriate treatment does not expose the woman to risk, it would seem reasonable clinical practice to commence a short course of empirical treatment with anticholinergic medication in cases where detrusor overactivity is suspected clinically, provided a midstream urine specimen is negative. If overactivity is present it should respond rapidly to such treatment.

Urodynamic investigation can be reserved for unresponsive cases where confirmation of the diagnosis is essential, both to avoid unnecessary continuation on unpleasant drugs and to exclude other pathology such as sensory urgency and stress incontinence where a different intervention will be required.

Women presenting with symptoms suggestive of detrusor overactivity without complications and who have yet to try medication do not require a urodynamic assessment. Cystometry is unlikely to alter their management significantly: if the urodynamic study fails to confirm detrusor overactivity and yet the history is highly suggestive, anticholinergic medication should not be withheld. They probably do have mild overactivity that has been missed: the laboratory test provides only an artificial 10–20 minute 'snapshot' and does not always replicate 'real life' events. For these women a trial of anticholinergics would be entirely appropriate.

Symptoms suggesting outlet obstruction

While symptoms of abnormal voiding in women are surprisingly common, outlet obstruction is rare. Symptoms of voiding dysfunction should initially be investigated with free urinary flows and post-void urinary residuals. If abnormal emptying is confirmed a full urodynamic assessment will help differentiate detrusor hypocontractility from outlet obstruction, which is sometimes seen in women with significant genitourinary prolapse, and rarely seen when there is loss of coordination between the sphincter and detrusor so that the sphincter does not relax appropriately (detrusor sphincter dyssynergia).

Women presenting with symptoms suggesting voiding problems require free urinary flows initially rather than a full urodynamic assessment. Voiding in a laboratory with catheter lines *in situ* is not conducive to replicating the 'normal' environment. Only if a free void in privacy and a post-void residual confirm abnormality should further assessment with cystometry be performed.

Neuropathic bladder

Women with neurological disease and lower urinary tract symptoms are at risk of neurogenic detrusor overactivity, low compliance and detrusor–sphincter dyssynergia. Of particular concern is the risk of upper tract damage when raised intravesical pressure results in upper tract dilatation and subsequent renal impairment. In these women a simultaneous assessment of anatomy (by videocystourethrography) and function (by pressure-flow studies) is essential. This known as video-urodynamics.

A full explanation of urodynamic investigation is beyond the scope of this text. It is however important that any clinician referring women for such tests has an understanding of what investigations are available and what the tests entail and can understand the information generated. The tests routinely performed include uroflowmetry, post-void residual measurement and cystometry. In addition, urethral pressure profilometry may be undertaken.

Uroflowmetry

The woman voids in privacy on a commode that incorporates a urinary flow meter, measuring voided volume over time. The flow pattern must be described when flow time and average flow rate are measured. A normal uroflow study consists of a total voided volume of more than 200 ml, voided over 15–20 seconds with a maximum flow rate of more than 20 ml per second and a smooth crescendo–decrescendo curve. Interpreting flows when voided volume is less than 200 ml is unreliable. A residual volume of more than 100 ml is considered as incomplete bladder emptying.

DEFINITIONS	
Voided volume	Total volume expelled via the urethra.
Maximum flow rate	Maximum measured value of the flow rate.
Average flow rate	Voided volume divided by flow time. The calculation of average flow rate is meaningful only if flow is continuous and without terminal dribbling.
Flow time	Time over which measurable flow actually occurs.
Residual urine	Volume of urine remaining in the bladder after a voluntary void.

CLINICAL INDICATIONS

Symptoms of dysfunctional voiding are nonspecific but if abnormal voiding is suspected it is important to investigate further with flows and post-void residuals. This is particularly important when investigating recurrent urinary tract infections or before commencing women with voiding symptoms on anticholinergic preparations for detrusor overactivity. Such medication can exacerbate inadequate voiding and large post-void residuals may lead to stasis, infection and renal damage. Furthermore, this is an essential preliminary test before proceeding with formal cystometry (see below), as many women find voiding in a laboratory environment with catheter lines *in situ* inhibiting; the results from the voiding phase of the cystometrogram should be interpreted with caution. If the uroflowmetry confirms abnormal voiding this suggests either obstruction or a poorly contracting detrusor muscle (cystometry will differentiate the two). These women are at an increased risk of voiding problems after retropubic surgery for urodynamic stress incontinence.

Cystometry

Cystometry aims to explain a clinical problem in pathophysiological terms by recording bladder pressure during filling and voiding. Detrusor overactivity is defined as 'a urodynamic observation characterised by involuntary detrusor contractions during the filling phase which may be spontaneous or provoked' and urodynamic stress incontinence is 'involuntary leakage of urine during filling cystometry during increased abdominal pressure, in the absence of a detrusor contraction'.[6]

The aim of cystometry is to reproduce the woman's symptoms and give a pathophysiological explanation of the woman's problem. The cystometrogram is used to measure the following features of bladder behaviour:

- capacity
- sensation
- compliance
- contractility
- urethral function.

During cystometry, the measurements shown in Table 4.1 are required (Figure 4.1). In addition, optional measurements and observations can be taken, as shown in the table. Figure 4.2 demonstrates loss of contrast medium from the bladder; incontinence occurred with coughing and the simultaneous pressure recording showed no detrusor activity. This therefore represents urodynamic stress incontinence.

The International Continence Society has done much over the years to standardise the methodology and interpretation of cystometry.[6] In

Table 4.1. Cystometry measurements

Measurement	Comments
Required	
Intravesical pressure (pves)	Usually measured with a urethral catheter
Intra-abdominal pressure (pabd)	Taken to indicate the pressure surrounding the bladder; usually estimated from rectal pressure
Detrusor pressure (pdet)	The component of intravesical pressure created by the active and passive forces in the bladder wall; it is derived from electronic subtraction of pabd from pves
Urine flow rate	Recording leakage during filling and flow during voiding
Volume infused	In order that bladder volume is known at any instant
Optional	
Urethral closure pressure (pura)	Derived from urethral pressure profilometry
Electromyography of pelvic floor or intra-urethral striated sphincter	
Videocystourethrography	When combined with pressure flow recordings known as videourodynamics

general, the woman should not be taking drugs that affect bladder function unless specified and variable factors that may affect results should be noted. These include the nature and temperature of the filling medium, whether the patient was supine, sitting or standing during the test, and the rate of artificial bladder filling. Fast bladder filling may produce significant urodynamic artefacts, particularly in neurological patients, and has previously been defined as fast filling (more than 100 ml/minute), medium filling (10–100 ml/minute) or slow filling (up to 10 ml/minute). It should, however, be remembered that the average physiological filling rate of the bladder is only 1 ml/minute, and therefore even the slow filling rate is not physiological except under extreme diuretic conditions. However, for the non-neurological patient a filling rate of 50–60 ml/minute during conventional cystometry appears to be a reasonable compromise, allowing realistic filling times and an apparent low incidence of artefacts.

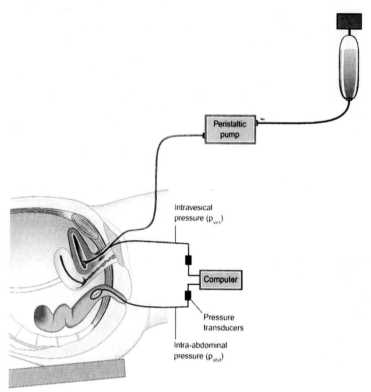

Figure 4.1 Insertion of three catheters; there are two in the bladder: one to fill the bladder and one to measure pressure; there is an additional catheter in the rectum to measure abdominal pressure

FILLING CYSTOMETRY

During the filling cystometrogram the following observations are made:

- capacity
- sensation
- compliance
- contractility
- urethral function.

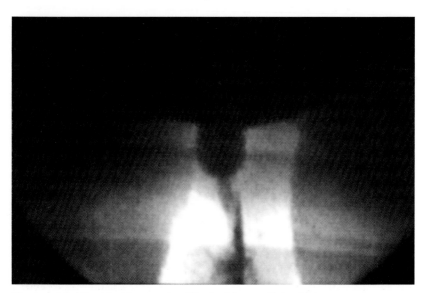

Figure 4.2 The bladder can be filled with a radiological contrast medium, allowing radiological imaging at the same time as performing pressure flow recording; this is known as videourodynamics. The figure demonstrates loss of contrast medium from the bladder; incontinence occurred with coughing and the simultaneous pressure recording showed no detrusor activity; this therefore represents urodynamic stress incontinence

Capacity

The volume infused during filling, and hence the calculated bladder volume, is measured. Assuming a normal rate of diuresis, natural filling should have a negligible contribution over the time span of a medium filling cystometrogram.

Sensation

The patient is asked to comment upon bladder sensation during filling. Terminology that can be used during the filling phase of the cystometrogram and that has been defined by the International Continence Society includes:

First sensation of bladder filling	The feeling the patient has, during during cystometry, when he or she first becomes aware of bladder filling, usually at approximately half capacity (150–200 ml).

First desire to void	The feeling that leads the patient to pass urine at the next convenient moment, although voiding can be delayed if necessary; commonly at 75% of capacity.
Strong desire to void	A persistent desire to void without fear of leakage, felt at capacity (300–600 ml).
Urgency	A sudden compelling desire to void, described particularly by patients with detrusor overactivity or inflammatory bladder conditions such as interstitial cystitis.
Maximum cystometric capacity	The volume at which the patient feels unable to delay micturition.

In practice, maximum cystometric capacity has little clinical application. All women attending for a cystometrogram are asked to complete a frequency/volume chart in the preceding week. From this and residual volume (negligible in most women), measured at the beginning of the cystometrogram study, functional bladder capacity can be calculated; this is 300–600 ml in most adults. Functional capacity is of much greater clinical relevance than maximum capacity and we would not recommend filling beyond functional capacity during the cystometrogram study. Overfilling yields no useful clinical data and there is a risk of precipitating poor voiding or even acute urinary retention due to overdistension of the bladder.

Compliance

This indicates the change in volume for a change in pressure. It is expressed as millilitres per centimetre of water and may be reduced if underlying pathology exists. During normal bladder filling little or no pressure change occurs; this is termed normal compliance. Rapid filling rates may alter this.

Contractility

In everyday life, the individual attempts to inhibit detrusor activity until in a position to void. Therefore, when the aims of the filling study have been achieved and when the patient has a normal desire to void, 'permission to void' is given. This moment is indicated on the urodynamic trace and all detrusor activity before this 'permission' is defined as involuntary detrusor activity.[6] If, during the filling phase, the

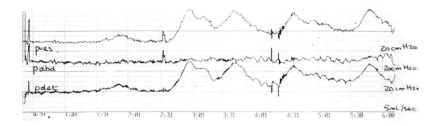

Figure 4.3 Top line shows a phasic increase in pressure within the bladder; middle line (pabd) does not show a similar rise in pressure; this therefore represents detrusor overactivity, which is clearly demonstrable on the bottom line (pdet); this being derived by subtracting abdominal pressure from intravesical pressure

bladder volume increases without a significant rise in pressure and with no involuntary contractions despite provocation the detrusor function is normal (stable). Detrusor overactivity is characterised by involuntary contractions during the filling phase which may be spontaneous or provoked. Any associated urinary leakage is called detrusor overactivity incontinence. Provocation may include rapid filling, alterations in posture and movement, coughing, tap running and other triggering procedures. Detrusor overactivity results in phasic contractions; this should be contrasted with altered compliance where the detrusor pressure rises gradually (Figure 4.3). The emphasis is on replicating symptoms, so in a patient with normal sensation pressure rises should be associated with urgency. If detrusor overactivity is present and there is objective evidence of a relevant neurological disorder the term neurogenic detrusor overactivity is used. When there is no defined cause it is termed idiopathic detrusor overactivity

Urethral function

The urethral closure mechanism during storage may be competent or incompetent. A normal urethral closure mechanism maintains a positive urethral closure pressure during bladder filling, even in the presence of increased abdominal pressure, although it may be overcome by detrusor overactivity. An incompetent urethral closure mechanism is defined as one which allows leakage of urine in the absence of a detrusor contraction.[6]

Urodynamic stress incontinence is noted during filling cystometry, and is defined as the involuntary leakage of urine during increased abdominal pressure, in the absence of a detrusor contraction.[6] To examine for this, we ask the woman to cough during the filling phase. Typically, such provocation will result in an instantaneous loss of urine. Examination of the subtracted pdet should confirm there to be no associated cough-induced instability before making the diagnosis of urodynamic stress incontinence.

Once the functional bladder capacity is reached, if stress incontinence has not been clearly demonstrated during the filling phase and the clinical history suggests this, the larger diameter filling catheter is removed, leaving the manometric tubing or electronic pressure sensing catheter *in situ* and the patient is asked to undertake a variety of provocative manoeuvres that can include coughing, squatting, heel bouncing and jumping. If urinary loss is observed, reference to the simultaneous pdet will elucidate whether the urethral closure is incompetent, or whether there was activity-provoked detrusor overactivity and associated detrusor overactivity incontinence.

VOIDING CYSTOMETRY

When filling cystometry has been performed the cystometrogram is completed by performing a voiding study. As previously discussed the filling catheter is removed before voiding to avoid unnecessary artefact through urethral obstruction. The intravesical and rectal pressure recording lines are left *in situ*, allowing the simultaneous measurement of detrusor pressure together with urine flow rate.

Normal voiding is achieved by voluntary initiation of a detrusor contraction which is sustained until the bladder is empty (Figure 4.4). The magnitude of the pressure rise depends on the degree of outlet resistance as well as the detrusor contraction itself. The normal male voids with a detrusor pressure of 20–40 cm H_2O but women have considerably lower pressures (10–25 cm H_2O), some voiding with excellent flows but little or no rise in pressure. This does not imply inadequate detrusor function, simply that the contraction is isotonic in the presence of low outlet resistance. The lower urethral resistance is reflected in the greater flow rates achieved by women. Detrusor activity is defined as inadequate if contractions are of insufficient magnitude or duration to effect bladder emptying in a normal time span in patients without significant outlet obstruction. If the detrusor pressure during voiding is low with low flow rates the detrusor is termed underactive (impaired contractility) and there may or may not be residual urine. If the detrusor shows no evidence of activity it is acontractile. Abdominal

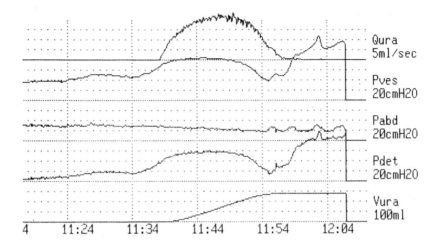

Figure 4.4 Top line shows a normal flow pattern; second line (pves) shows a rise in intravesical pressure; third line (pabd) shows no rise in intra-abdominal pressure. The patient therefore has voided by initiating a detrusor contraction; this represents normal voiding function

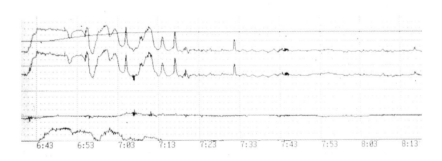

Figure 4.5 Flow is depicted on the bottom line; this is reduced and intermittent. The top line represents intravesical pressure and the second line represents abdominal pressure. In this trace, the phasic increases in pressure are similar in both intravesical and intra-abdominal lines. The third line, derived by subtracting pabd from pdet, represents detrusor pressure; this line is flat, there is no contraction of the detrusor muscle and this patient is emptying her bladder by straining

straining should not be required if the detrusor is functioning normally (Figure 4.5).

The urinary flow recorded during voiding cystometry should be correlated with the detrusor activity. In most circumstances in adults a voided volume of less than 100 ml cannot be interpreted reliably while flow rates obtained above 500 ml cystometric capacity may also be low, perhaps owing to bladder decompensation. Outlet obstruction should cause a low to normal flow with raised detrusor pressure when compared with normal controls. Most patients will be able to void during the study, but some will be inhibited by the laboratory situation. An abnormal flow or residual during voiding cystometry does therefore not in itself indicate a functional abnormality if subsequent free flow rates performed in privacy with residual urine assessment indicate normality.

It should be remembered that urodynamic studies are invasive and, although extremely safe, complications such as urinary tract infections occasionally occur. Furthermore patients find the test undignified and may find catheterisation uncomfortable. Therefore, to avoid unnecessary anxiety, morbidity and expense it is important to select women appropriately for cystometry. This requires an understanding of the test's clinical indications (see above).

AMBULATORY STUDIES

The controversy surrounding artificial filling rates has led to the development of natural fill cystometry and long-term ambulatory monitoring. These systems use microtip pressure transducers to record rectal and bladder pressure; the signals are digitised and transferred to solid state memory. If the machine incorporates an integrated voiding channel, data from a flowmeter can be stored in the memory allowing simultaneous recordings of urinary flow and detrusor activity. First desire to void, urgency, micturition and subjective leakage can be recorded by the woman in the memory using coded event marker buttons. Studies may last up to 24–48 hours, if required, depending on the portable memory capacity. During the course of the study, the woman can perform tasks that normally provoke symptoms such as hand washing, running and carrying heavy bags. One of the limitations of the technique is the difficulty of simultaneously recording urinary incontinence; during conventional cystometry this is simply done by the supervising clinician by direct inspection of the urethral meatus. During ambulatory studies one usually relies on confirming incontinence by measuring perineal pad weight gain and timing the incontinent episodes by asking the woman to press an event marker button when leakage occurs. This is subjective and therefore inherently less reliable.

Ambulatory urodynamics may prove to be a significant development. Data derived from artificial filling cystometry may be unreliable for a number of reasons: the filling rate is nonphysiological; the test requires catheterisation, is of a relatively short duration and is performed in a physically confined clinical setting, often in full view of strangers. Ambulatory monitoring overcomes some of these limitations. It does appear more sensitive in the detection of detrusor overactivity and incontinence than conventional cystometry.[7-9] In women with incontinence not seen on conventional cystometry, ambulatory monitoring recording over two or three micturition cycles will allow correlation of the woman's symptoms (recorded by a coded event marker), changes in detrusor pressure and episodes of urinary leakage. Using this technique, we find ambulatory monitoring particularly useful for defining whether leakage is due to detrusor overactivity or an incompetent urethral closure mechanism in women with objective loss on pad testing and a normal conventional urodynamic study. It is also of considerable help in those women with symptoms of frequency, urgency and urge incontinence and a normal conventional cystometry.[10]

Urethral pressure profilometry

To maintain continence, urethral pressure must remain higher than intravesical pressure. Withdrawing a microtip catheter through the urethral sphincter at a predefined speed allows the urethral pressure curve to be measured. Data from the profile so produced includes:

- **maximum urethral pressure**, which is the maximum pressure of the measured profile

- **maximum urethral closure pressure** (MUCP), which is the maximum difference between the urethral pressure and the intravesical pressure

- **functional profile length**, which is the length of the urethra along which the urethral pressure exceeds intravesical pressure (Figures 4.6 and 4.7).

Theoretically, urethral pressure profilometry should differentiate between stress incontinence secondary to urethral hypermobility (these women should have good intrinsic sphincter function, hence a reasonable urethral closure pressure) and that secondary to intrinsic sphincter deficiency. This should help the clinician decide on

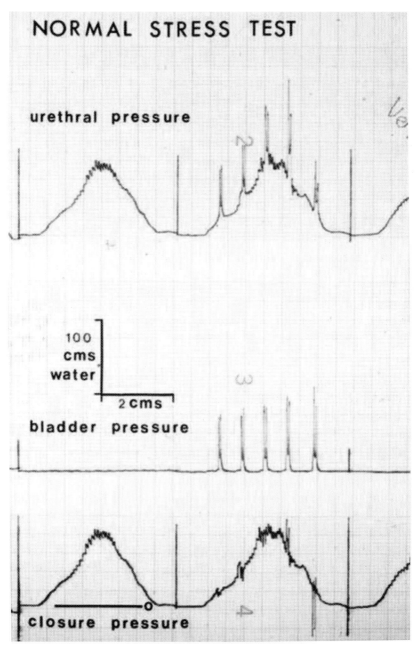

Figure 4.6 A normal urethral pressure profile; the maximal urethral closure pressure is over 60 cm water and when the patient coughs, pressure is transmitted to the proximal urethra; this should be compared with Figure 4.7

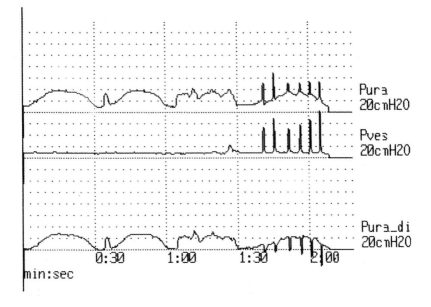

Figure 4.7 The urethral pressure here is much lower than in Figure 4.6. When the patient coughs there is suboptimal pressure transmission; coughing causes pressure rise in the bladder (pves), which is not transmitted well to the urethra (pura)

appropriate surgery (for example, a colposuspension would intuitively seem appropriate in the woman with hypermobility, while the woman with a well-supported bladder neck but a low MUCP has intrinsic sphincter deficiency and is unlikely to benefit from such surgery). Clinically, however, there is a considerable range of MUCP values. Hypermobility can be determined from clinical examination and most centres in the UK therefore do not routinely perform urethral pressure profilometry. It has been suggested that women with a low urethral closure pressure (less than 20 cm H_2O) have increased surgical failure following retropubic procedures,[11] and many clinicians would recommend alternative surgery such as a urethral sling in such cases. There is no robust data to support such a philosophy, and it has been disputed;[12] no randomised trial has ever been undertaken to explore this hypothesis.

Perineal pad testing

A simple way of measuring urine loss is by weighing a perineal pad, before and after use. A one-hour test, performed with a comfortably full bladder during usual daily activities, results in a mean pad weight increase of less than 1 g in women with normal urinary control. Loss of more than 2 g is generally regarded as a positive result. This one-hour test has been reported as reliable and reproducible.[13] The test is clinically useful when conventional urodynamic testing fails to confirm the symptom of urinary incontinence; if pad testing confirms urinary loss further investigation with ambulatory urodynamic testing is appropriate and may elucidate the cause of the urinary incontinence.

Diagnostic cystourethroscopy

Diagnostic cystourethroscopy can be performed using a rigid or flexible cystoscope, with or without anaesthesia. Water is the preferred distending medium used during cystoscopy. Cystoscopes with several differently angled lenses are available (0°, 30° and 70°) and this allows visualisation of all of the lower urinary tract; the 70° scope will usually be required to adequately inspect the anterolateral walls of the bladder and to visualise the trigone and bladder base if a cystourethrocoele is present. Comment should be made on the appearance of the urethra, bladder mucosa, trigone and ureteric orifices. If bladder filling symptoms are present the clinician should also comment on volume of fluid infused (with or without anaesthesia; under anaesthetic a normally compliant bladder should easily accept more than 800 ml of fluid).

Diagnostic cystourethroscopy is indicated in cases of recurrent urinary tract infection, haematuria, bladder pain and suspected lower urinary tract injury. Endoscopic examination is also frequently indicated peri-operatively, to assess urethral wall coaptation during urethral injection, to exclude urethral or bladder perforation when surgical instruments have been passed blindly retropubically (e.g. Stamey or 'TVT' needles), to assess elevation of the bladder neck and to facilitate safe insertion of suprapubic catheters.

CYSTOSCOPIC FINDINGS

Normal

The bladder mucosa is normally pale pink with a smooth surface. The trigone is granular and thick with a villous contour. Histology of this area often shows squamous metaplasia. The trigone and the ureteric

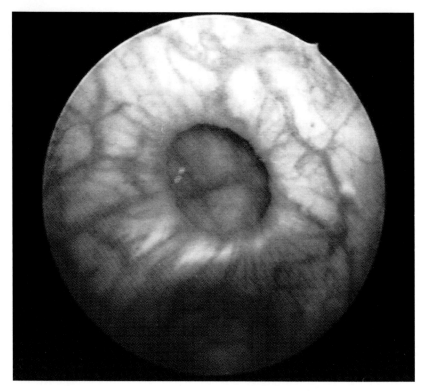

Figure 4.8 Cystoscopic appearance of a bladder diverticulum

openings are seen on the posterior bladder wall past the bladder neck (see Figure 2.8).

Abnormal

The abnormalities may be mucosal or structural. Pathology seen may include diverticula (urethral or bladder) (Figure 4.8), foreign bodies, calculi, carcinoma, inflammation (infective, radiation or interstitial cystitis) (Figure 4.9) and fistulae. The most common mucosal abnormality is cystitis. In cases of suspected interstitial cystitis, it is important to perform the procedure under general anaesthetic. The bladder is distended and drained and then a second-look cystoscopy is performed. The mucosa may show glomerulations or petechial haemorrhages in interstitial cystitis (Figure 4.10). A guided biopsy should be taken to confirm the diagnosis.

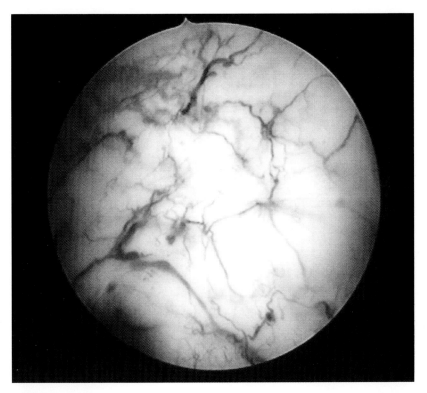

Figure 4.9 Cystoscopic appearance of the bladder following irradiation; the tissue is much paler than normal and contains an abnormal vascular pattern

Imaging

The lower urinary tract can often be investigated adequately without imaging. Imaging is much more commonly required in suspected disease of the upper renal tract and as such is the preserve of urologists and renal physicians, and beyond the scope of this book. However, there are conditions gynaecologists may encounter where imaging is required. These conditions include:

- recurrent urinary tract infections

- haematuria

- urethral diverticula, which need to be differentiated from paraurethral cysts

- suspected ureteric injury

- suspected urethral or vesical fistulae.

RECURRENT URINARY TRACT INFECTIONS

Ultrasound or contrast computed tomography (CT) scan of the bladder and kidneys may exclude incomplete bladder emptying, congenital anomalies and ureteric reflux with cortical scarring.

HAEMATURIA

As well as cystourethrography, the upper renal tract needs investigating for calculi with plain radiographs and for renal tumours with ultrasound or CT scanning.

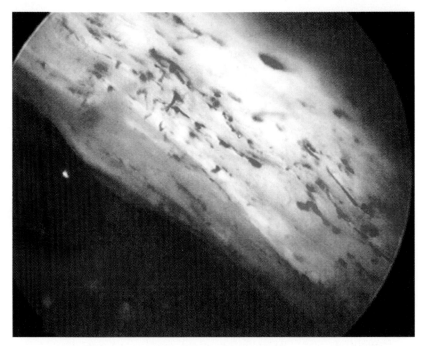

Figure 4.10 Cystoscopic appearance of interstitial cystitis; the bladder mucosa has split during bladder distension and there are areas of haemorrhage

URETHRAL DIVERTICULA

Urethral diverticula need to be differentiated from paraurethral cysts. Magnetic resonance imaging (MRI) is the investigation of choice. A cyst can be simply excised without damaging the urethra while excising a diverticulum runs the risk of creating a urethrovesical fistula. Such surgery should be undertaken by a surgeon with experience of urethral reconstruction.

SUSPECTED URETERIC INJURY

If acute ureteric obstruction is suspected, renal ultrasound is the initial investigation of choice. Any dilatation of the upper tract collecting system should then be investigated further with contrast urography; the contrast either being injected intravenously and excreted via the kidneys or instilled up the ureter by retrograde fill. These are also the initial investigations of choice where division of the ureter is suspected.

SUSPECTED URETHRAL OR VESICAL FISTULAE

If nothing can be seen on cystourethroscopy and fistulae are suspected, further investigation with MRI scanning and contrast cysto-urethrography may be diagnostic.

References

1. Kaufman JM. Urodynamics in stress incontinence. *J Urol* 1979;**122**:778–82.
2. Hastie KJ, Moisey CU. Are urodynamics necessary in female patients presenting with stress incontinence? *Br J Urol* 1989;**63**:155–6.
3. James M, Jackson S, Shepherd A, Abrams P. Pure stress leakage symptomatology: is it safe to discount detrusor instability? *Br J Obstet Gynaecol* 1999;**106**:1255–8.
4. Jarvis GJ, Hall S, Stamp S, *et al.* An assessment of urodynamic examination in incontinent women. *Br J Obstet Gynaecol* 1980;**87**:893–6.
5. Cardozo LD, Stanton SL, Williams JE. Detrusor instability following surgery for genuine stress incontinence. *Br J Urol* 1979;**51**:204–7.
6. Abrams P, Cardozo L, Fall M, Griffiths D, Rosier P, Ulmsten U, *et al.* The standardisation or terminology of lower urinary tract function: Report from the Standardisation Subcommittee of the International Continence Society. *Neurouro Urodyn* 2002;**21**:167–78.
7. Swithinbank L, James M, Shepherd A, Abrams P. Role of ambulatory urodynamic monitoring in clinical urological practice. *Neurourol Urodyn* 1999;**18**:215–22.
8. Salvatore S, Khullar V, Cardozo L, Anders K, Zocchi G, Soligo M. Evaluating ambulatory urodynamics: a prospective study in asymptomatic women. *BJOG* 2001;**108**:107–11.
9. Heslington K, Hilton P. Ambulatory monitoring and conventional cystometry in asymptomatic female volunteers. *Br J Obstet Gynaecol* 1996;**103**:434–41.
10. Radley SC, Rosario DJ, Chapple CR, Farkas AG. Conventional and ambulatory urodynamic findings in women with symptoms suggestive of bladder overactivity. *J Urol* 2001;**166**:2253–6.

11. McGuire EJ. Urodynamic findings in patients after failure of stress incontinence operations. *Prog Clin Biol Res* 1981;**78**:351–60.
12. Maher CF, Dwyer PL, Carey MP, Moran PA. Colposuspension or sling for low urethral pressure stress incontinence? *Int Urogynecol J Pelvic Floor Dysfunction* 1999;**10**:384–9.
13. Sutherst J, Brown M, Shawer M. Assessing the severity of urinary incontinence in women by weighing perineal pads. *Lancet* 1981;**I**:1128–113.

5   Urinary stress incontinence

Introduction

Stress incontinence is the complaint of involuntary leakage on effort or exertion, or on sneezing or coughing,[1] and suggests a problem with urethral competence. Urodynamic stress incontinence is noted during filling cystometry and is defined as the involuntary leakage of urine during increased abdominal pressure, in the absence of a detrusor contraction.[1] Prevalence figures for urinary incontinence vary widely. It is thought that urinary loss secondary to urodynamic stress incontinence is slightly more common than that secondary to detrusor overactivity. These two conditions account for the vast majority of female incontinence in the developed world, although globally fistulae from obstructed labour is another major cause.

Aetiology

The aetiology of stress incontinence is undoubtedly multifactorial. Some women appear to have a congenital predisposition, possibly because of inherently weak collagenous connective tissue.[2] Childbirth has always been thought to be a major contributory factor for many women. Vaginal delivery has for some time been known to cause denervation of the pelvic floor.[3] However, it is only since 1999 that prospective studies have confirmed a correlation between vaginal delivery and subsequent urinary incontinence,[4] and no long-term prospective data are currently available. Whether the menopause and subsequent oestrogen deficiency is implicated or not is contentious. Some prevalence data suggest an increase in urinary incontinence around the perimenopause but other studies refute this.[5-7] Anything that places chronic strain on the pelvic floor may also predispose to urinary stress incontinence; such factors include constipation, obesity and chronic cough.

Conservative management

Treatment should initially be conservative. As discussed in Chapter 3, conservative treatment can usually be implemented without recourse to urodynamic assessment. It is therefore the symptom of stress incontinence that is being treated initially.

LIFESTYLE ADJUSTMENTS

Encourage cessation of smoking, treat chronic cough conditions, advise regarding weight reduction and rectify exacerbating conditions such as constipation.

PELVIC FLOOR EXERCISES

Pelvic floor exercises were first described by Kegel in 1948 and are best taught by a physiotherapist. The aims are to promote patient awareness and improve contractility and coordination of pelvic floor muscles.

The pelvic floor musculature is made up of predominantly slow twitch fibres, which are involved in posture, and a smaller element of fast twitch fibres, which are used during exertion such as coughing. Slow twitch fibres are trained with long sustained repetitive pelvic floor exercises whereas fast twitch fibres are trained with fast powerful contractions.

An assessment of pelvic floor strength should be made in all women with urinary stress incontinence. Vaginal examination is performed to palpate the levator ani muscles. Pelvic floor strength is graded 0 to 5 on a modified Oxford scale and endurance (or length of time of maximum contraction and number of repeated contractions) is also recorded. If the muscle is weak an exercise regimen is then introduced, concentrating on both contraction strength and muscle endurance. Regimens vary: three sets of 8–12 slow velocity maximal contractions sustained for 6–8 seconds each per day would be common but many physiotherapists will individualise a programme to the particular woman rather than being too prescriptive. If improvement has not been observed within 3–4 months further treatment is unlikely to be beneficial.

Additional techniques are frequently employed by physiotherapists to maximise pelvic floor contractility. 'Biofeedback' is a term referring to the use of a device to convert the effect of a pelvic floor contraction into a visual or auditory response signal. It allows patients and health professionals to observe improvement in an objective manner. One such device is a perineometer (Figure 5.1). This is placed within the vagina and records pelvic floor contractile strength numerically. It will however also register raised vaginal pressure secondary to a Valsalva manoeuvre and so cannot be used in isolation for pelvic floor muscle training. Pudendal nerve stimulation with an electrode can be useful if the initial pelvic floor contraction is weak, the woman having little voluntary

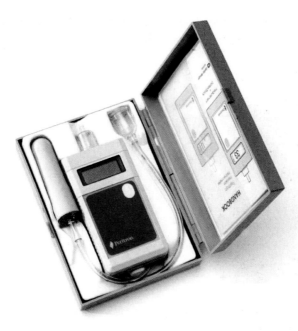

Figure 5.1 Perineometer; this is placed within the vagina and records pelvic floor contractile strength numerically

pelvic floor contraction (Figure 5.2). A woman can use the device for 20 minutes a day at home and adjust the strength of stimulation herself. Weighted vaginal cones can help women to identify the muscles of the pelvic floor. Cones of increasing weight (20–90 g) are inserted into the vagina and the woman trains her muscles to prevent the cone falling out (Figure 5.3). These have been popular since they were introduced in 1985 and subjective improvement rates can be as high as 70%.[8] They have the advantage of not requiring direct physiotherapy supervision. Some professionals have reservations about the long isometric contractions required with vaginal cones and fear injury may result due to overuse. However, there is little evidence that this is a problem in practice.

Pelvic floor exercises will be appropriate first line treatment for most women. However, a proportion will not benefit and additional investigation and treatment should not be delayed. Women unlikely to benefit include those in whom muscle strength and endurance is already excellent and those who are not able to master the technique or have insufficient motivation.

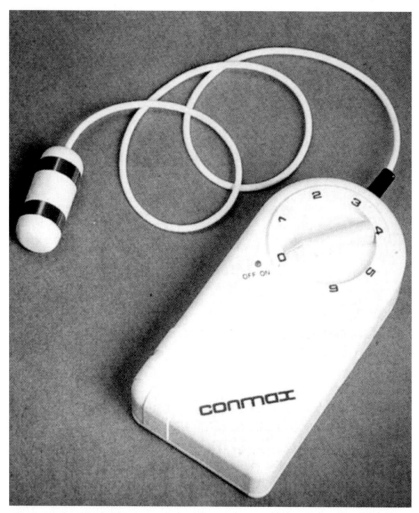

Figure 5.2 Pudendal nerve stimulator with an electrode can be useful

Pelvic floor exercises have been compared with no treatment for incontinent women in two randomised controlled trials.[9] Women performing pelvic floor exercises were more likely to be dry or mildly incontinent (61%) than those receiving no treatment (3%). Exercises need to be continued on a long-term basis to prevent recurrence of symptoms.

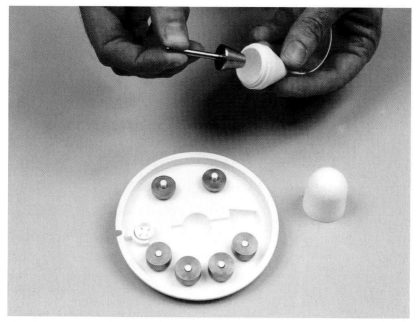

Figure 5.3 Vaginal cones

MECHANICAL CONTINENCE DEVICES

These may be appropriate while women await definitive treatment or in women who do not feel sufficiently inconvenienced by their symptoms to consider invasive therapy, for example if leakage only occurs with specific activities such as aerobics or vigorous sports.

Devices may be vaginal or urethral. Vaginal devices probably exert their effect by compressing the urethra transvaginally or by supporting the urethra and bladder neck. Examples include foam pessaries and sponge tampons. Urethral devices are either intraurethral, providing occlusion, or are applied to the external urethral meatus, forming a cap. Their main disadvantage is that removal is necessary each time the woman wishes to micturate (Figure 5.4).

Pharmacotherapy

Theoretically, several classes of drug could be beneficial in the treatment of urinary stress incontinence.

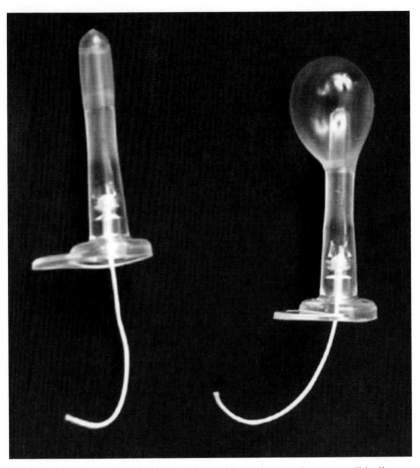

Figure 5.4 Urethral plug; once inserted into the urethra, a small balloon at the tip of the plug keeps the device in place

The urethral sphincter is under autonomic control with sympathetic alpha-adrenergic receptors causing contraction of the urethral sphincter. However, alpha-agonists appear to have limited benefit: there is little evidence of efficacy from randomised controlled trials. Oestrogens have been proposed as a treatment of stress incontinence; many women feel their incontinence gets worse or commences around the time of the menopause. However, trials do not support their use,[10,11] although there is some evidence that oestrogens used in conjunction with alpha-agonists may be beneficial.[12] Other compounds are being developed and assessed. At present attention is focusing on a potent selective norepinephrine and serotonin reuptake inhibitor (duloxetine). Animal work suggests it increases neural activity to the external urethral sphincter via a central action at Onuf's nucleus in the spinal cord. Clinical studies have confirmed efficacy in treating stress incontinence.[13] This and other drugs provide a realistic expectation that urinary stress incontinence may become medically treatable in the near future.

Surgical treatment of urodynamic stress incontinence

Before considering any surgical intervention the clinician should make a definitive diagnosis of stress incontinence with a urodynamic assessment. The reasons for this are three-fold. Firstly, history and examination are not reliable: the woman may have cough-provoked detrusor overactivity rather than sphincter weakness. Secondly, surgery can exacerbate pre-existing detrusor overactivity. Thirdly, surgery can cause retention; this risk is significantly higher if urodynamic studies reveal preoperative detrusor hypocontractility or outflow obstruction. Without a prior urodynamic assessment the clinician will not know whether surgery is appropriate and will not be able to counsel women adequately on potential postoperative complications.

The choice of surgical procedure should be made according to the underlying pathophysiology of the stress incontinence. Surgical procedures generally rectify either bladder neck hypermobility or intrinsic sphincter deficiency even though the two may coexist in the same woman. Differentiating hypermobility from the well-supported bladder neck is critical when considering the suitability of certain operations. Urethral hypermobility is treated by operations that support the bladder neck. The most common procedure would be a colposuspension although needle suspensions, sling procedures and anterior colporrhaphy will also support the bladder neck. Intrinsic sphincter deficiency is treated with procedures to improve sphincter function and urethral closure. Commonly bulking agents are injected into the periurethra or slings are inserted. In extreme cases artificial sphincters can be implanted. When the bladder neck is well supported a colposuspension is unlikely to be beneficial and would be an inappropriate intervention.

In practical terms, slings can be used to treat stress incontinence, whether secondary to hypermobility or intrinsic sphincter deficiency. As new techniques such as tension free vaginal tape (TVT), a form of urethral sling, become widely adopted, differentiating hypermobility from intrinsic sphincter deficiency becomes less clinically important.

When deciding on surgery a balance must be made between efficacy and potential complications. For example, a woman may choose periurethral injections, accepting the procedure has mediocre efficacy but aware there is a low risk of long-term urinary retention. Surgical procedures should also be tailored to individual women's clinical features.

FACTORS THAT NEED TO BE TAKEN INTO ACCOUNT IN ANY DECISION ABOUT SURGERY

- Is the woman fit enough to withstand general or spinal anaesthesia or is a local anaesthetic required?

- Is the woman going to be physically active? If so the surgery will have to withstand more stress.

- Obesity increases the risk with any surgical procedure; this is particularly pertinent when contemplating deep pelvic surgery. Haemorrhage may be life-threatening if vision and access are poor.

- Is it likely that the procedure will have to last 5 years or 50 years?

- Has the woman finished childbearing? If not definitive major continence surgery is best avoided.

- If postoperative retention occurs how would the woman cope psychologically with self-catheterisation? Is she physically able to perform this? Elderly women with unsteady hands and poor vision are less likely to cope with the technique.

- Is there hypermobility or intrinsic sphincter deficiency?

- If either detrusor overactivity or voiding dysfunction is present on the preoperative urodynamic assessment the clinician may wish to avoid potentially obstructive surgery.

- If concurrent prolapse is present a procedure may need to be selected that will reduce it or avoid exacerbating it further. For example, a colposuspension will reduce a low cystocele, but will exacerbate a rectocele.

Over 150 surgical treatments for urodynamic stress incontinence have been described and few have been subject to large prospective randomised controlled trials. Outcomes are therefore difficult to compare. Different populations may have been operated on: for example, co-morbidity, previous failed continence surgery and absence of a preoperative urodynamic assessment will all adversely affect outcomes without necessarily reflecting an inadequate surgical procedure. Furthermore, methods of measuring 'success' vary in different studies and the duration of postoperative follow-up differ. Bearing these caveats in mind, some frequently performed surgical procedures have been subjected to meta-analyses and systematic review to establish their success rates and complications.[14]

Informed consent for a surgical procedure should include a detailed discussion regarding the risks and benefits of the proposed operation. Furthermore, so that the woman can make an informed choice about the surgery, she should also be aware of the risks and benefits of other procedures. Anyone contemplating continence surgery should be told the procedure's failure rate, together with the risks of *de novo* detrusor overactivity and urinary retention, both of which may be permanent. Figures may vary from surgeon to surgeon, and where possible an individual unit's results should be presented. Where this is not available, data may need to be presented from published meta-analyses.[14,15]

The following is not intended to be an exhaustive list of available continence procedures, but does include those most commonly in use.

RETROPUBIC SUSPENSIONS

The Marshall–Marchetti–Krantz procedure

First described in 1949, the Marshall–Marchetti–Krantz procedure used to be the most widely used suprapubic incontinence operation. Via a low transverse suprapubic incision, sutures are placed between periurethral tissues and the periosteum of the posterior aspect of the superior pubic ramus. The mean success rate in the meta-analysis performed by Jarvis in 1994 is 89.5% for a first procedure.[14] Complications include osteitis pubis in 2.5–5.0% and urethrovaginal fistulae in 0.3%. Long-term voiding difficulty affects 11.0–12.5% and the incidence of *de novo* detrusor overactivity is thought to be in the region of 11%. Compared with the Burch colposuspension, the risk of postoperative prolapse is thought to be insignificant because there is little elevation of the anterior vaginal wall which predisposes to later enterocele formation. However, for the same reason the Marshall–Marchetti–Krantz procedure cannot be used to treat a cystocele.

The Marshall–Marchetti–Krantz procedure has largely been superseded by the Burch colposuspension. This is partly because of the technical difficulty of retaining sutures in the periosteum and partly because of the significant risk of osteitis pubis, which is difficult to treat and may become chronic.

The Burch colposuspension

First described in 1961, the Burch colposuspension can be used to treat stress incontinence when bladder neck hypermobility is present. As in the Marshall–Marchetti–Krantz procedure, the retropubic space is entered through a low transverse suprapubic incision. Sutures are placed between the paravaginal fascia and ipsilateral ileopectineal ligament (Cooper's ligament) at the level of the bladder neck. The surgery aims to elevate and support the hypermobile bladder neck (Figure 5.5). Low cystocele can also be corrected. Colposuspension deviates the vaginal axis anteriorly, so any pre-existing enterocele or rectocele will be exacerbated and may occur *de novo*.

The Burch colposuspension has been modified by many and, although often called the 'gold standard' operation, we have never seen two surgeons perform the operation in an identical manner. Common variables include: suture material (absorbable or permanent, mono-filament or multibraided), suture tension (some try to approximate the vagina to the ileopectineal ligament while others use minimal tension) and suture position (which varies on the vagina from mid-urethral level to above the bladder neck, and on the pubis from near the symphyseal midline to lateral near the obturator foramen).

In theory, absorbable sutures will increase the risk of failure, while excessive elevation and medial suture placement increases the risk of urethral compression with consequent outlet obstruction and voiding difficulty. This emphasises the importance of auditing individual surgeons' outcomes so that techniques can be modified if necessary.

Overall, meta-analysis of published data suggests that the efficacy of the Burch colposuspension as a primary procedure is 89.8% and as a repeat procedure is 82.5%.

Complications include haemorrhage and injury to the bladder or ureter. Rarely, the ureter may be kinked if sutures are placed too laterally. There is a significant risk of postoperative vaginal prolapse, most notably enterocele formation which affects up to 18%. *De novo* detrusor overactivity affects between 10 and 25%, although some of this may be pre-existing overactivity that was missed with conventional preoperative cystometry. Immediate voiding difficulty occurs in 12–25% although only 2% are affected more than six months postoperatively. Often these can be predicted preoperatively: women with preoperative low urinary flow rates (less than 12ml/sec) or high voiding pressures (>15 cm H_2O) are at greatest risk.

Laparoscopic colposuspension

First described in 1991 by Vaincaille, a number of variations of technique

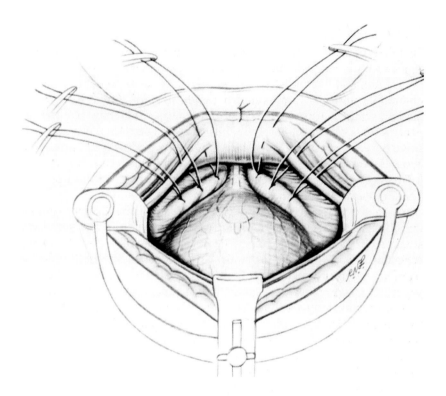

Figure 5.5 Burch colposuspension showing suturing of the vagina at the level of bladder neck to the iliopectineal ligament

have been described, with surgeons using a variety of suture materials, clips and meshes. When done well, laparoscopic surgery appears to precisely replicate the open procedure and affords a better magnified view of the surgical field. The surgery however is technically demanding and requires considerable laparoscopic expertise. As for conventional colposuspension, the results will be operator dependent and the outcome of a UK multicentre randomised controlled trial comparing open with laparoscopic colposuspension is currently awaited. Data comparing efficacy, complication rates and recovery times are required before deciding whether this technique is worth the additional expense, both in terms of laparoscopic equipment and additional theatre time.

Needle suspension procedures

First described in 1959 by Pereyra, these have subsequently been modified by a number of surgeons, most notably Stamey and Raz. The paraurethral tissue or bladder neck is suspended from the anterior abdominal wall by passing long nylon sutures retropubically and attaching the suture to paraurethral tissue with helical sutures or paraurethral pledgets. Suspension is easy to perform with minimal dissection, low intraoperative blood loss and a short operating time. Women require only a short hospital stay and morbidity is low.

On occasion, after endoscopic bladder neck suspension, sutures have been thought to migrate to the inside of the bladder. A significant number of women will suffer persistent wound pain; Jarvis[14] reported this to be as high as 27%. Sinus formation can occur at the site of the sutures. Infection of the buffers may be as high as 13%. Detrusor overactivity and voiding disorder occur in up to 6%. Short-term success rates were initially high, with Stamey reporting a 91% cure rate at 6 months.[16] However, success is much lower in the long term. At 10 years the continence rate is only 6–10%[17] and as a consequence few centres now perform this operation.

ANTERIOR COLPORRHAPHY

Surgical treatment for anterior vaginal prolapse was first described in 1888 by Schultz. It was modified by Kelly who, in order to treat urinary incontinence, plicated the paravesical tissue at the bladder neck and excised a portion of the vaginal wall. Complication rates are low but can include injury to the bladder or urethra and haemorrhage. In the long term there may be recurrent prolapse, urinary incontinence and rarely urethral stricture. The incidence of voiding disorders postoperatively is low but postoperative *de novo* detrusor overactivity may occur in up to 8%. There is relatively little postoperative pain allowing early mobilisation and discharge from hospital.

As a first procedure for the treatment of stress incontinence the success rate is only 67.8%.[14] Bergman and Elia reported a one-year success rate of 63% with a dramatic fall to 37% at five years.[18] In the same study the colposuspension was shown to be more effective at one and five years with success rates of 89% and 82% respectively.

Therefore, although widely used in the treatment of vaginal prolapse, it is no longer commonly used as a first line treatment for stress incontinence. The high recurrence rate for urinary incontinence after anterior colporrhaphy, and the scarring of the vagina jeopardising any subsequent surgery such as colposuspension, add weight to the argument that anterior colporrhaphy should be reserved for the treatment of prolapse alone. However, as for injectable therapy, mediocre efficacy needs to be offset against the lower complication rates when compared with other procedures such as colposuspension, and the procedure may still have a role in the elderly woman with stress incontinence and concurrent cystocele.

Slings

Material can be slung beneath the urethra or bladder neck and anchored, often to a point on the anterior abdominal wall. The mechanism of action has been debated. The slings can be inserted under tension, partially obstructing the urethra. Such insertion causes a high incidence of postoperative voiding dysfunction and bladder filling symptoms. More recently, slings have been inserted under minimal tension. These probably work by allowing effective transmission of increased intra-abdominal pressure around the urethra, providing support and passive resistance rather than urethral compression.

Slings can be used for the treatment of stress incontinence secondary to either hypermobility or intrinsic sphincter deficiency. In the UK, hypermobility has commonly been treated with colposuspension, sling procedures being reserved for the treatment of recurrent stress incontinence after previous failed surgery, particularly if there is scarring and fixing of the urethra with poor urethral sphincter closure. The advent of minimally invasive techniques such as the polypropylene sling (tension-free vaginal tape) have, however, changed many clinicians' practice and slings are now commonly inserted as primary procedures.

Procedures using the vaginal, abdominal and abdominal–vaginal routes have been described. It would seem that no route is superior. Instead of anchoring to the anterior abdominal wall, some techniques describe bone anchoring or anchoring to Cooper's ligaments. Some synthetic slings require no attachment; presumably they fibrose to surrounding tissue.

Initially, slings were made of autologous tissue such as pyramidalis muscle, rectus fascia with pyramidalis and even gracilis muscle. In 1942, Aldridge described a combined abdominal–vaginal sling procedure using thin horizontal strips of rectus fascia mobilised using a Pfannenstiel incision. The fascia was left attached at the medial border and brought through the cave of Retzius and endopelvic fascia to sit on either side of the urethra, united in the midline beneath the urethra at the level of the bladder neck.

Subsequently, slings have been developed from extrinsic tissue. Such allogenic slings have included cadaveric fascia lata and dura mater, and animal tissue such as porcine dermis. There is an inherent risk of infection, although manufacturing techniques which reduce antigenicity and sterilise appear to render tissue safe. Efficacy, however, is questionable; absorption and shrinkage can occur.

More recently, plastic synthetic materials have been employed. Materials include polyethylene (Mersilene®, Ethicon), polypropylene (Prolene®, Ethicon) and polytetrafluoroethylene (Gore-Tex®). There is a risk of local tissue reaction, persistent infection and also urethral erosion and fistula formation. These risks vary considerably depending upon the material used and the characteristics of the mesh weave, such as pore size.

Overall, when results from traditional slings were subjected to meta-analysis,[14] objective cure rates of 93.9% for primary procedures and 86.1% for recurrent procedures were obtained. However, as discussed with colposuspension, results from meta-analysis can be misleading when differing sling types and operative techniques are combined. Ideally, surgeons should be able to quote their own outcome data.

Voiding disorders occur in 12.8% (range 2–37%)[14] and these can sometimes be treated with urethral dilation in the immediate postoperative period. Occasionally, the sling can be incised. Intermittent self-catheterisation is required by 1.5–7.8% in the long term.[19] *De novo* detrusor overactivity occurs in 16.6% (range 4–29%).[14] Erosion of the sling through the urethra or vagina occurs predominantly with synthetic sling materials. The incidence is approximately 1–6% with the exception of Gore-Tex where it is much higher.[20]

TENSION-FREE VAGINAL TAPE

Tension-free vaginal tape (TVT), a transvaginal sling inserted at the level of the mid-urethra, was first described in Sweden in 1995[21] and has now become established practice in the UK. It has altered clinical practice to such a degree that many surgeons are no longer performing other surgery, such as colposuspension. A combination of minimal tension (the term 'tension-free' is a misnomer), a mesh made of polypropylene and mid-urethral positioning appears to confer much lower complication rates than seen with previous slings.

The procedure is minimally invasive and was first described for use under local anaesthesia, with some centres inserting it as a daycase procedure. However, voiding problems can occur and regional or general anaesthesia is preferred by many, particularly where more difficult surgery is anticipated. The sling is inserted transvaginally, aiming to provide support at mid-urethral level. A trocar is passed retropubically (Figures 5.6, 5.7, 5.8 and 5.9) bilaterally and cystoscopy should be performed after the insertion of each trocar to detect

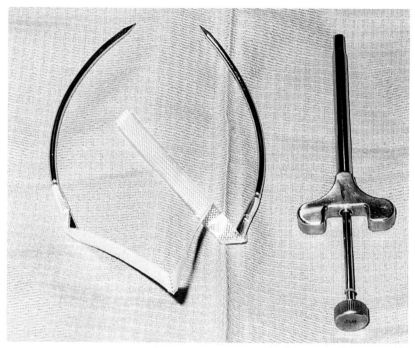

Figure 5.6 A TVT urethral sling

perforation of the bladder. A 70-degree cystoscope is essential as anterolateral bladder wall perforation may be missed if a 30-degree or 0-degree scope is used. If the bladder has been traumatised, the trocar is removed and inserted again. Once the tape is positioned, tension is applied while the woman coughs. Variables between surgeons include the mode of anaesthesia, the Valsalva manoeuvre used to provoke leakage and the volume of fluid in the bladder when attempting to provoke leakage. Some surgeons will tension the tape until the woman is completely dry. However, we now recognise that the risk of postoperative retention is similar to colposuspension and, furthermore, the polypropylene tape is thought to shrink by 20% *in vivo*. Therefore, many now leave the woman slightly incontinent with coughing perioperatively; they are usually dry postoperatively.

A multicentre randomised controlled trial comparing TVT with colposuspension has confirmed similar efficacy at 12 months.[22] Although overall cure rates for both colposuspension and TVT were similar, individual centres' cure rates differed markedly for both procedures,

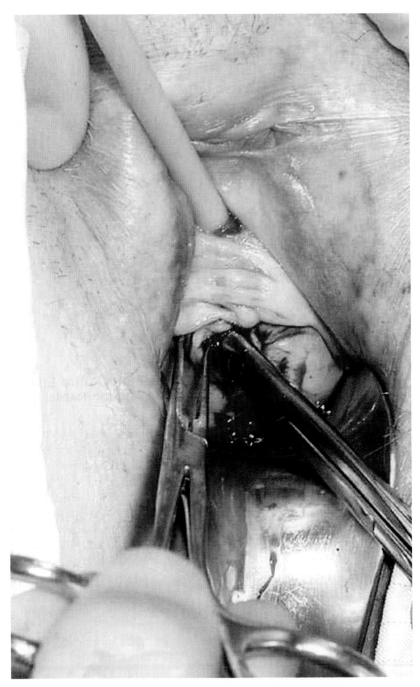

Figure 5.7 Careful dissection around the mid-urethra

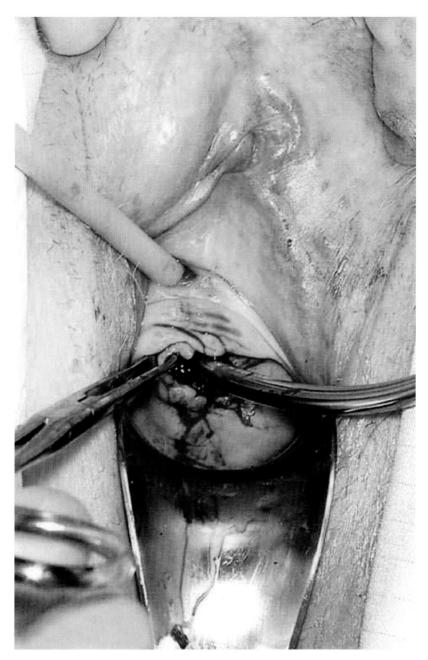

Figure 5.8 Insertion of the trocar at the level of the mid-urethra; note the use of a urethral catheter to deviate the urethra away from the surgical field

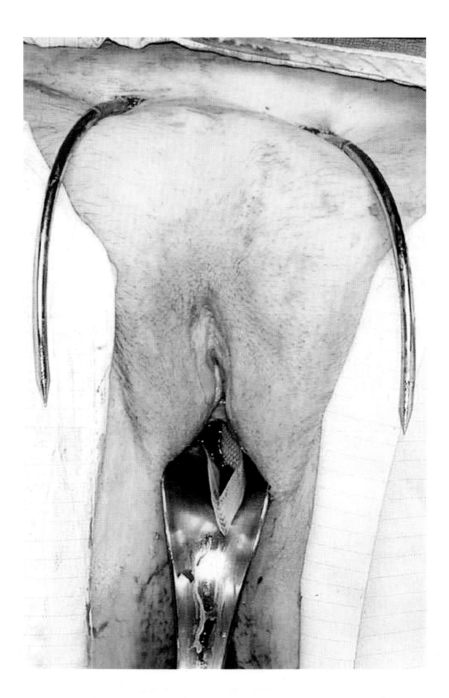

Figure 5.9 The trocar is passed retropubically bilaterally

emphasising the need for individual surgeons to audit their own outcomes rather than rely on nationally or internationally quoted figures. When compared with the Burch colposuspension, the TVT has lower estimated blood loss, operation duration, hospitalisation and analgesia requirement. It is the minimally invasive nature of the technique and the quicker recovery phase that appeals to many surgeons. Furthermore, because vaginal anatomy is not distorted the procedure does not, unlike colposuspension, predispose to rectocele. However, there is a higher risk of bladder injury with TVT – 9% (compared with 2% with colposuspension) and as high as 19% in women who have had previous surgery for urodynamic stress incontinence. Bladder puncture tends to occur more frequently at the beginning of the learning curve. There do not seem to be long-term sequelae of recognised bladder perforation. If the bladder has been perforated a Foley catheter is recommended for 24–72 hours and 5 days of antibiotics should be prescribed. Other recognised complications include injury to the obturator and iliac vessels. The tape may become infected and perioperative antibiotics should be given. Long-term follow-up is not yet available although Ulmsten et al.[21] have reported 4-year follow-up data. Tape erosion into both the vagina and the urethra have been described and although the erosion rate is currently thought to be low it is not known whether the incidence will rise with time.

Periurethral bulking injection

Periurethral injection with a bulking agent is thought to achieve continence by improving apposition of the urethral epithelium. Various materials have been injected. Autologous fat and Teflon® have been used in the past. However, Teflon produced a granulomatous reaction with fibrosis; it also migrated to distant organs such as brain and lung. Autologous fat was rapidly phagocytosed and long-term results were consequently disappointing. Injection has also been complicated by fat embolism. Currently, the two most commonly used injectables are collagen (Contigen®, Bard Inc.) and silicone rubber (Macroplastique®, Uroplasty BV).

Glutaraldehyde cross-linked bovine collagen (GAX collagen) is a sterile purified form of bovine dermal collagen stabilised by cross-linking. As it is allergenic in 3% a skin test is done four weeks before surgery. It produces a local inflammatory response and some reports suggest the GAX collagen can be replaced with endogenous collagen. Migration of the collagen particles does not seem to occur. Macroplastique is a popular injectable composed of micronised silicone rubber particles suspended in a nonsilicone carrier gel. Once injected, the carrier gel is removed by the host inflammatory response and replaced with collagen and the silicone becomes encapsulated in fibrin. Migration does not seem to occur; this is probably because of the particle size. There have been no published trials comparing different materials for bladder neck injection.

Other newer injectables are becoming available but are not yet widely researched. Extracts of bovine collagen, carbon coated silicone particles, bone and ceramic materials are under investigation.

Injections are usually given with cystoscopic guidance although urethral guides have been developed to allow blind insertion of Macroplastique in the outpatient setting. Injection can be performed under local anaesthesia, regional block or general anaesthetic (Figure 5.10a,b). The technique is minimally invasive and has an extremely low complication rate; retention is rare and most patients can go home the same day. It is unlikely to exacerbate detrusor overactivity.

Reported cure rates vary but may be as low as 7% for objective cure. The success rate of periurethral bladder neck injection in the treatment of primary urodynamic stress incontinence was 45.5% according to Jarvis's meta-analysis in 1994 and 57.8% in recurrent stress incontinence.[14] Efficacy is often short-lasting, particularly if a reabsorbable product such as collagen is used, and reinjection is frequently required.

While the injectable materials are expensive and the results mediocre, the procedure has a low complication rate and a quick recovery phase. This makes the technique particularly suitable for the frail elderly. Other minimally invasive techniques such as TVT may also be suitable for this group but injectables have a much lower risk of precipitating retention. This is particularly pertinent if there is pre-existing poor detrusor function and the woman has poor hand–eye coordination which makes self-catheterisation unfeasible.

Treatment for intractable urodynamic stress incontinence

End-stage procedures are indicated after multiple failed continence procedures and where there are congenital abnormalities and neuropathic disorders such as spina bifida, multiple sclerosis and spinal cord injury.

ARTIFICIAL SPHINCTERS

Since it was first used in 1973, the artificial urinary sphincter has been developed. It is made of silastic and consists of a variable-sized occlusive cuff placed around the bladder neck which can be inflated and deflated

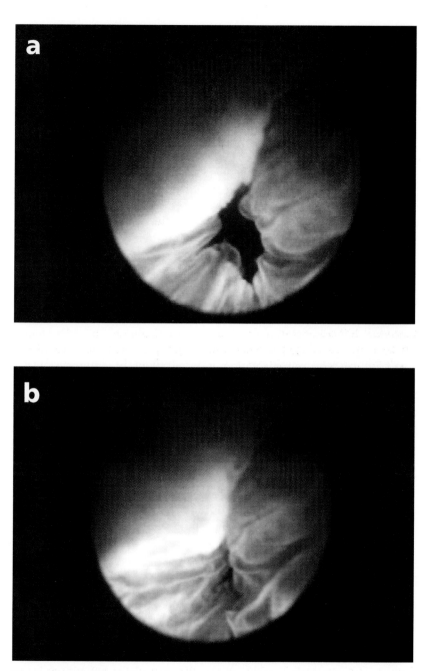

Figure 5.10a & b Collagen has been injected into the urethral mucosa at 7 o'clock, leading to apposition at the urethral mucosa

to maintain continence and void as required. The reservoir for the cuff is inserted beneath the rectus and the pump mechanism is implanted into one of the labia majora.

Short-term success is high with maintained improvement in 90% at five years, although almost one-third will require revision surgery. The expense of the device and a high complication rate limit use: urethral erosion occurs in up to 30% and infection in up to 20% of cases.

URINARY DIVERSION

Permanent urinary diversion is occasionally indicated in women with intractable incontinence. Such procedures are continent diversions which involve the use or creation of a reservoir within the body to store urine. A surface sphincter is created which is then catheterised to empty the reservoir making the urethra and even the bladder redundant.

The Kock principle creates a continence reservoir from small intestine; a pouch is fashioned from a segment of ileum. At either end the bowel is intussuscepted to create a narrowing or gut nipple valve which reduces reflux and efflux. One nipple intussusception is attached to the anterior abdominal wall where it acts as a sphincter enabling the pouch to be emptied by catheterisation. The other nipple intussusception is used for ureteric reimplantation. Complications of enterocystoplasty include fluid and electrolyte disturbance, stones, infections, malignant change and mucus production. This technique would be reserved for women where the bladder has to be substituted because of disease. Where the bladder wall remains healthy but the woman has intractable incontinence, the Mitrofanoff principle allows the bladder to continue to be used as the continence reservoir. The urethra is made redundant by the creation of an outflow tract at the anterior abdominal wall. The appendix is used to connect the bladder to the anterior abdominal wall. The caecal end is attached to the outside and the distal end is tunnelled into the anterolateral bladder wall creating a flutter valve. The bladder is emptied by means of a catheter.

Catheterisation may be required on a long-term basis in women with intractable incontinence, usually in the frail elderly with multiple concomitant pathologies that preclude alternative management. Many such women and their carers find permanent catheterisation a better option than continuous severe incontinence. Catheters may be urethral or suprapubic. Urethral catheters should be selected with the narrowest appropriate lumen. In the long term, this may need to be slightly larger (up to 16 g) as there is a risk of encrustation of the catheter. Silicone catheters and plastic or latex catheters coated with silicone reduce encrustation. Female catheters are 20–25 cm and can be used with discreet leg bags worn under clothing. If a permanent indwelling catheter is required suprapubic drainage is often preferable, as this does not irritate the urethra or trigone, and the urethra cannot be traumatised by the woman pulling on her catheter.

Complications of catheterisation include urinary tract infection. Colonisation of the foreign body may make eradication difficult and antibiotics are only indicated if the urinary infection is symptomatic. Bypassing of urine around the catheter is a common problem. Changing the catheter will be helpful if there is lumen obstruction from mucus or encrustation. If, however, bypassing continues it may be due to detrusor overactivity and can be treated with anticholinergics.

INCONTINENCE PADS

Incontinence pads may be a temporary or a permanent aid for those with urinary or faecal incontinence. Women who use them vary from those with extremely mild symptoms who wear a small pad for reassurance to those with intractable severe leakage who would otherwise require a catheter. As a consequence the type of pad required varies enormously. Superabsorbent hydrogels are covered by material that allows penetration of urine but prevents backflow to the surface of the pad.

References

1   Abrams P, Cardozo L, Fall M, Griffiths D, Rosier P, Ulmsten U, *et al.* The standardisation or terminology of lower urinary tract function: Report from the Standardisation Subcommittee of the International Continence Society. *Neurourol Urodyn* 2002;21:167–78.
2   Keane DP, Sims TJ, Abrams P, Bailey AJ. Analysis of collagen status in premenopausal nulliparous females with genuine stress incontinence. *Br J Obstet Gynaecol* 1997;104:994–8.
3   Snooks SJ, Swash M, Henry MM, Setchell ME. Injury to innervation of pelvic floor sphincter musculature in childbirth. *Lancet* 1984;ii:546–50.
4   Chaliha C, Kalia V, Stanton SL, Monga A, Sultan H. Antenatal prediction of postpartum urinary and faecal incontinence. *Obstet Gynecol* 1999;689–94.
5   Jolleys JV. Reported prevalence of urinary incontinence in women in general practice. *BMJ* 1988;296:1300–02.
6   Thomas TM, Plymat KR, Blannin J. Prevalence of urinary incontinence. *BMJ* 1980;281:1243.
7   Versi E, Cardozo L, Studd J, Brincat M, Cooper D. Urinary disorders and the menopause. *Journal of the North American Menopause Society* 1995;2(2):89–95.
8   Peattie AB, Plevnik S, Stanton SL. Vaginal cones: a conservative method of treating genuine stress incontinence. *Br J Obstet Gynaecol* 1988;95:1049–53.
9   Berghmans LCM, Hendriks HJM, Bo K, *et al.* Conservative treatment of stress urinary incontinence in women: a systematic review of randomised controlled trials. *Br J Urol* 1998;82:181–91.
10   Fantl A, Cardozo L, Eckberg J, McClish D. Estrogen therapy in the management of urinary incontinence in postmenopausal women: a meta analysis. *Obstet Gynecol*

1994;83:12–18.
11 Jackson S, Sheperd A, Brookes S, Abrams P. The effect of oestrogen supplementation on postmenopausal urinary stress incontinence: a double blind placebo-controlled trial. *Br J Obstet Gynaecol* 1999;106:711–18.
12 Cardozo LD, Kelleher CJ. Sex hormones, the menopause and urinary problems. *Gynecol Endocrinol* 1995;9:75–84.
13 Van Kerrebroeck P, Abrams P, Lange R, Slack M, Wyndaele JJ, Yalcin I, *et al.* Duloxetine versus placebo in the treatment of European and Canadian women with stress urinary incontinence. *BJOG* 2004;111:249–57.
14 Jarvis GJ. Surgery for genuine stress incontinence. *Br J Obstet Gynaecol* 1994;101:371–4.
15 Black NA, Downs SH. The effectiveness of surgery for stress incontinence in women: a systematic review. *Br J Urol* 1996;78:497–510.
16. Schaeffer AJ, Stamey TA. Endoscopic suspension of vesical neck for urinary incontinence. *Urology* 1984;23:484–94.
17 Chaliha C, Stanton SL. Urethral Sphincter Incompetence. In: *Clinical Urogynaecology*. 2nd ed. London: Churchill Livingstone;2000. p. 201–17.
18 Bergman A, Elia G. Three surgical procedures for GSI; 5 year follow up of a prospective randomised study. *Am J Obstet Gynecol* 1995;173:66–71.
19 Ghonheim G, Shaaban A. Suburethral slings for the treatment of stress urinary incontinence. *Int Urogynaecol J* 1994;5:228–39.
20 Rezapour M, Ulmsten U. Tension Free Vaginal Tape (TVT) in women with recurrent stress urinary incontinence: a long term follow up. *Int Urogynecol J Pelvic Floor Dysfunct* 2001;12 Suppl 2:S9–11.
21 Ulmsten U, Henriksson L, Johnson P, Varhos G. An ambulatory surgical procedure under local anaesthesia for treatment of female urinary incontinence. *Int Urogynaecol J Pelvic Floor Dysfunct* 1996;7:81–6.
22 Ward K, Hilton P. Prospective multicentre randomised controlled trial of tension free vaginal tape and colposuspension as primary treatment for stress incontinence. *BMJ* 2002;325:7355;67–70.

6   Detrusor overactivity

Introduction

We gain bladder control as young children and from this time onwards a healthy bladder is controlled by the central nervous system. The detrusor will not contract until it is convenient to initiate a void. This contraction is initiated at the level of the cerebral cortex. When detrusor overactivity is present, however, the detrusor contracts spontaneously during the filling phase of the micturition cycle, when micturition would normally be inhibited. The true incidence of this condition is unknown; it is possible that we all exhibit detrusor overactivity on occasions. For example, many 'healthy' people will have symptoms of urinary urgency when the weather is cold, when they have drunk strong coffee or when they put their key in the front door with a full bladder. In some people, this condition causes great distress and can manifest as severe urinary frequency with urgency. There may be associated urge urinary incontinence; this can be particularly distressing as the bladder may empty completely off an unstable detrusor contraction.

Definitions

Detrusor overactivity is defined as 'a urodynamic observation characterised by involuntary detrusor contractions during the filling phase which may be spontaneous or provoked' (e.g. by rapid bladder filling, alterations of posture, the sound of running taps).[1] It is apparent from this definition that, as there has to be objective evidence of a detrusor contraction, detrusor overactivity can be diagnosed only after a urodynamic study. It is neither necessary nor desirable to investigate all women presenting with symptoms of frequency, urgency and urge incontinence with a urodynamic study. When the history is typical, one can usually presume that there is underlying detrusor overactivity and treat empirically for 1–2 months. Urodynamics can be reserved for those in whom empirical treatment fails.

Urgency, with or without urge incontinence, usually with frequency and nocturia, can be described as 'overactive bladder syndrome'.[1] This symptom combination suggests detrusor overactivity but can be caused by other forms of urethrovesical dysfunction. The term can be used after urinary infection and other obvious pathology has been excluded. Therefore, before empirical treatment the woman should complete a urinary diary and have urine tested for blood and infection to exclude factors such as malignancy, untreated diabetes and polydipsia.

Aetiology

It is no surprise, given the wide range of people who are thought to display detrusor overactivity, that this is not a homogenous disease with a single cause. In a minority of sufferers, there is a disturbance of the nervous control mechanisms and when there is objective evidence of a relevant neurological disorder in association with detrusor overactivity diagnosed on urodynamic testing, the term 'neurogenic detrusor overactivity' is used. However, the vast majority of sufferers have no associated neurological disease and this condition is commonly termed 'idiopathic detrusor overactivity'. In clinical practice, the extent of neurological examination and investigation varies. If there are no overt neurological symptoms most clinicians would not investigate further, for example with magnetic resonance imaging (MRI). It is likely that a complete neurological assessment would result in some idiopathic cases being reclassified as neurogenic. As the name implies, the underlying aetiology of idiopathic detrusor overactivity is unknown. Sometimes obstruction is implicated: men may see a resolution of both bladder-filling symptoms (such as frequency and urgency) and urodynamically proven detrusor overactivity after relieving prostatic obstruction. In women, potentially obstructive continence surgery can result in *de novo* detrusor overactivity. The risk of this appears to vary according to the continence procedure chosen, with the more obstructive operations conferring the highest risk. The quoted incidence of *de novo* overactivity is 1% after anterior colporrhaphy, 6% after endoscopic bladder neck surgery and 10% after colposuspension and suburethral sling procedures.[2] The majority of women with detrusor overactivity do not, however, have any bladder outlet obstruction and other factors must be implicated that are currently imperfectly understood.

Treatment

As the pathophysiology of the disease is poorly understood, the cause cannot yet be treated and management aims to suppress the symptoms rather than alter the disease process itself. The natural history of idiopathic detrusor overactivity is completely unknown. In many people, this will be a remitting disease and symptom suppression may result in longer-term resolution. Treatment may therefore be either short- or long-term, depending on the individual.

BEHAVIOUR MODIFICATION

Behaviour modification, such as reducing fluid intake if the urinary diary suggests this is excessive, and cutting caffeinated products out of the diet will often have a dramatic effect. Simple advice such as this may be all that is required to cure frequency and urgency.

BLADDER TRAINING

The three main components of bladder training are patient education, timed voiding with systematic delay of voiding and positive reinforcement. The woman is asked to resist the sensation of urgency and void according to a timetable. She is told that she is not allowed to use the toilet until the next scheduled time of void. Initially, bladder drill insisted on inpatient treatment to ensure strict adherence to the protocol but most centres would now treat women as outpatients, using self-completed urinary diaries to monitor the times of voids. Continence rates of up to 90% have been reported[3] but cure rates in most centres would be considerably lower than this. Relapse is common: after 3 years, published success rates fall to 40% or less.[4]

OTHER NONPHARMACEUTICAL THERAPIES

Hypnotherapy has been shown to be of value: women voided less frequently and held greater volumes of urine: 50% were reported to become symptom free although treatment needed to continue indefinitely to maintain benefit.[5] Other treatments that have been reported to be of benefit include psychotherapy, acupuncture and electrostimulation.

PHARMACOTHERAPY

Pharmacological suppression of detrusor overactivity is the most widely used treatment for this condition, athough tolerance is limited by adverse effects. The wide variety of drugs available is testament to the drawbacks of each drug.

Antimuscarinics

Anticholinergics are the mainstay for pharmacological treatment of detrusor overactivity. The most commonly prescribed treatment for the overactive bladder in the UK is currently oxybutynin, although some of the second-generation products are increasingly widely used. Oxybutynin has three actions: antimuscarinic, direct muscle relaxant and local anaesthetic. Its efficacy has been shown in both open and controlled trials.[6,7] The main drawback of high-dose (5 mg three times daily) oxybutynin has been the incidence of adverse effects: up to 40% withdraw from treatment within 3 months[8] and 80% will suffer adverse effects such as dry mouth and blurred vision. A modified-release preparation with once daily administration is now available. This preparation retains the efficacy of the standard-release form with up to 40% fewer reported adverse effects.[9]

Tolterodine is a second-generation product that appears to have functional selectivity for muscarinic receptors in the bladder over those in the salivary glands. In doses of 2 mg twice daily, tolterodine results in a reduction in frequency, urgency and the number of incontinence episodes. Like oxybutynin, tolterodine is now also available in a once daily slow-release form which may help minimise potential adverse effects.[10,11]

Tricyclic antidepressants have anticholinergic as well as alpha-adrenergic properties, thereby inhibiting bladder contractions and increasing urethral tone. Daytime and nocturnal symptoms have been reduced in 74% and 60% patients, respectively.[12] Imipramine 10–25 mg one to three times daily is the most commonly used tricyclic antidepressant.

Propiverine, trospium chloride, solifenacin and darifenacin are more recent additions to the list of available drugs.[13] These preparations have not been investigated as extensively as the older products but appear to be useful additions.

Anticholinergic adverse effects can occur with any of the above compounds and include dry mouth, dizziness, blurred vision, constipation, nausea and insomnia. Some may tolerate particular preparations better than others and the clinician may need to try a number of the above before finding one that suits the individual. Dosage may need to be titrated against clinical efficacy and the adverse effect profile, although the newer drugs are in general better tolerated than conventional quick release oxybutynin, so reducing the need for dose titration.

Anticholinergics are contraindicated in people with narrow-angle glaucoma and myasthenia gravis.

Oestrogens

Some women develop bladder-filling symptoms after the menopause. There is evidence, both anecdotal and from uncontrolled trials, that oestrogen supplementation is therapeutic. There is, however, remarkably little robust evidence to support this premise: controlled trials have largely looked at an unselected population with urinary incontinence of mixed aetiology or have concentrated on urinary stress incontinence.

Other drugs

Calcium antagonists have in the past been used to suppress bladder-filling symptoms. The most commonly prescribed preparation was terodiline, but this was withdrawn from the market because of a possible association with cardiac arrhythmias and there has been a reluctance by pharmaceutical companies to develop this field further.

Potassium channel openers are being investigated but, at present, adverse effects limit use and no preparation currently has a licence.

SURGICAL TREATMENT

Surgery is recommended for intractable detrusor overactivity only when medical and behavioural therapy has failed. Commonly, it is the woman severely affected by neuropathic disease with concomitant detrusor overactivity who requires surgery, although women with severe idiopathic detrusor overactivity may also be suitable. The mainstay of surgical management is augmentation cystoplasty, although cystodistension and bladder denervation have been used and new developments such as neuromodulation and botulinum toxin injection may offer hope for the future.

Prolonged cystodistension

The term 'cystodistension' covers a variety of procedures, such as stretching the bladder at the time of cystoscopy using gravitational hydrostatic pressure, instilling fluid under manometric pressure (usually midway between diastolic and systolic pressure) for 5 minutes, and inflating an intravesical hydrostatic balloon for 2–6 hours at a pressure midway between systolic and diastolic blood pressure. The complications of cystodistension include bladder rupture, and prolonged distension can result in bladder atony, probably as a result of ischaemic nerve damage reducing detrusor contractility. Complications and poor efficacy limit use of the procedure. Morbidity of 20% and patient satisfaction of 27% have been reported.[14]

Denervation procedures

The rationale is that reduction in motor efferent activity gives rise to reduced detrusor contractility and hence reduction in unwanted detrusor contractions. Bladder denervation can be accomplished by peripheral and central procedures. Techniques described have included selective sacral neurectomy, subtrigonal phenol injection into the parasympathetic pelvic plexus, and transvaginal transection of the inferior hypogastric plexus as it approaches the bladder base. Complications and poor long-term efficacy again limit the applicability of denervation procedures.

Augmentation cystoplasty

This is the current gold standard surgical therapy. When severe overactivity is present, the high intravesical pressures generated cause debilitating urge incontinence and also risk ureteric reflux with reflux nephropathy. Cystoplasty involves splitting the bladder and sewing in a compliant segment of tissue. Usually autologous tissue is used – commonly a loop of ileum on a vascular pedicle – although other tissues include caecum and ureter (if there is already a terminally damaged kidney). Such surgery physically increases bladder capacity and, more importantly, the elastic properties of the autologous segment prevent high intravesical pressure rises when unstable detrusor contractions occur. This protects the upper renal tract from reflux and cures urge incontinence. Because bladder contractility is compromised patients are at high risk of subsequent retention: they should be taught to self-catheterise preoperatively. When bowel has been used to augment the bladder the mucosa continues to secrete mucus: there is a risk of mucus retention, stone formation and malignant change in the autologous tissue. Regular check cystoscopies are indicated.

RECENT ADVANCES

Detrusor myectomy

The complications of cystoplasty with autologous tissue are described above. Myectomy entails removing detrusor muscle from the dome of the bladder, leaving mucosa intact. The surgery is intuitively attractive: the urine remains in contact with normal bladder mucosa, a compliant 'pouch' is formed that theoretically confers the advantages of the cystoplasty, while potential complications such as mucus secretion and malignant change are circumvented. Patients are still likely to require self-catheterisation and, as the technique is relatively new, the long-term benefits are currently unknown.

Electrical stimulation and neuromodulation

Detrusor overactivity can be treated by influencing the sacral micturition reflex arc. Techniques described include implanting electrodes either around the whole nerve root or around the ventral roots in conjunction with dorsal rhizotomy (cutting the dorsal roots). Postulated mechanisms for action include stimulating the tone within the urethral sphincter which may have a suppressive effect on the detrusor. Paradoxically, improvements in detrusor contractility and bladder emptying have also been reported. The destructive nature of the surgery has limited applicability to all but the women most severely affected by neuropathic disease and more recently attention has focused on sacral nerve root stimulation without rhizotomy. Results are currently preliminary and the true place of neuromodulation has yet to be fully determined.

Botulinum toxin

Botulinum toxin paralyses muscle. It has been pioneered within plastic surgery, paralysis of the periorbital muscles reducing facial wrinkles. Other applications have been proposed and there is some preliminary evidence that injecting into the detrusor inhibits symptoms of bladder overactivity. Efficacy is short-lived: injections probably require repetition every 3 months and we await more clinical data.[15]

KEY POINTS

- Detrusor overactivity is a common condition causing considerable distress.

- Symptoms include frequency, urgency and nocturia, with or without urge incontinence.

- Exclude intravesical pathology in women who have haematuria and bladder pain.

- Treat with bladder training, fluid management and anticholinergics.

- If there is no symptomatic relief, perform urodynamics to exclude neurogenic causes and determine detrusor overactivity.

- Pharmacotherapy includes oxybutynin, tolterodine and other tricyclic antidepressants.

- Surgery is reserved for those with intractable detrusor overactivity that does not respond to pharmacotherapy.

References

1. Abrams P, Cardozo L, Fall M, Griffiths D, Rosier P, Ulmsten U, *et al.* The standardisation or terminology of lower urinary tract function: report from the Standardisation Subcommittee of the International Continence Society. *Neurourol Urodyn* 2002;21:167–78.
2. Jarvis GJ. The management of urinary incontinence. In: Jarvis GJ, editor. *Obstetrics and Gynaecology*. Oxford: Oxford University Press; 1994. p. 260–99.
3. Jarvis GJ, Millar DM. Controlled trial of bladder drill for idiopathic detrusor instability. *BMJ* 1980;281:1322–3.
4. Holmes DM, Stone AR, Barry PR, *et al.* Bladder training – 3 years on. *Br J Urol* 1983;55:660–64.
5. Freeman RM, Guthrie KA, Baxby K. Hypnotherapy for idiopathic detrusor instability: a two year review. *BMJ* 1985;290:286.
6. Moisey CU, Stephenson TP, Brendler CB. The urodynamic and subjective result of treatment of detrusor instability with oxybutynin. *Br J Urol* 1980;52:472–5.
7. Cardozo LD, Cooper D, Versi E. Oxybutynin chloride in the management of idiopathic detrusor instability. *Neurourol Urodyn* 1997;6:256–7.
8. Chapple CR. Muscarinic receptor antagonists in the treatment of overactive bladder. *Urology* 2000;55 (5A Suppl):33–46.
9. Anderson RU, Mobley D, Blank B, *et al.* Once daily controlled versus immediate release oxybutynin chloride for urge urinary incontinence. *J Urol* 1999;161:1809–12.
10. Van Kerrebroeck P, Kreder K, Jonas U, *et al.* Tolterodine once daily: superior efficacy and tolerability in the treatment of overactive bladder. *Urology* 2001;57:414–21.
11. Abrams P, Freeman R, Anderstrom C, Mattiasson A. Tolterodine, a new antimuscarinic agent: as effective but better tolerated than oxybutynin in patients with overactive bladder. *Br J Urol* 1998;81:801–10.
12. Castledon CM, Duffin HM, Gulati RS. Double blind study of imipramine and placebo for incontinence due to bladder instability. *Age Ageing* 1986;15:299–303.
13. Kershen RT, Hsieh M. Preview of new drugs for overactive bladder and incontinence: darifenacin, solifenacin, trospium, and duloxetine. *Curr Urol Rep* 2004 Oct;5:359–67.
14. McCahy PJ, Styles RA. Prolonged bladder distension: experience in the treatment of detrusor overactivity and interstitial cystitis. *Eur Urol* 1995;28:325–7.
15. Harper M, Fowler CJ, Dasgupta P. Botulinism toxin and its application in the lower urinary tract. *BJU Int* 2004;93:702–6.

7 Haematuria

Haematuria may originate from any site along the urinary tract and may signify underlying pathology. It may be microscopic or macroscopic but investigation is similar.

Prevalence

Using dipstick testing the prevalence of haematuria is 2–16%. Dipstick testing is sensitive but not specific and it may detect physiological amounts of blood in the urine. Therefore, while a useful screening test, it should be confirmed with microscopy. Microscopic haematuria is present if there are three or more red blood cells per high power field in urinary sediment from two of three freshly voided, clean-catch midstream urine specimens.[1] The prevalence of haematuria on microscopy is between 1% and 5%.

Aetiology

In women under 50 years with microscopic haematuria 2–10% will have urinary tract pathology. This is most commonly stones, specific infections and nephritis. Urinary tract malignancy is rare below 40 years. Approximately 10–20% of women over 50 years with microscopic haematuria will have significant urinary tract pathology which is often malignancy and this risk is increased if frank haematuria is present.[2]

Management

CLINICAL HISTORY

Recent menstruation or sexual trauma may indicate another source of the bleeding and the clinician should try to differentiate haematuria from vaginal and rectal bleeding. Urinary frequency or dysuria suggests a urinary tract infection, which is the most common cause of haematuria in young women. Urinary tract calculi may be associated with pain and glomerulonephritis or nephropathy may be secondary to a recent upper respiratory tract infection, rash or oedema. Medication may be responsible: nonsteroidal anti-inflammatory drugs can cause papillary necrosis while cyclophosphamide and danazol can cause haemorrhagic cystitis. Anticoagulants should not cause haematuria unless the woman is over-anticoagulated. Some food pigments and drugs such as beetroot and rifampicin can mimic macroscopic haematuria.

Bladder cancer classically presents as painless frank haematuria. Other risk factors for significant disease include age over 40 years, smoking, exposure to dyes or chemicals and a history of pelvic irradiation.

INVESTIGATION

Microscopy

Haematuria on dipstick should always be confirmed by microscopy on a midstream sample of urine before further evaluation is undertaken. Urine microscopy can provide additional information about the morphology of the red blood cells. Dysmorphic red blood cells are usually of glomerular origin, whereas normal red blood cells are usually from the lower urinary tract. Red cell casts are virtually pathognomonic for glomerular disease.

Urine culture

This is vital to exclude urinary tract infection. Haematuria should never be attributed to infection unless there is a positive urine culture. In this situation a repeat urine specimen should be tested 6 weeks after treatment to exclude continuing microscopic haematuria.[3]

Biochemistry

Urine should be tested for proteinuria, which may be a sign of renal pathology or an extra renal medical disorder. In the presence of significant proteinuria (greater than 1+ on dipstick or greater than 1 g/24 hours on biochemical analysis) serum urea, creatinine and electrolytes should be measured.

Urine cytology

Cytology can detect transitional cell carcinoma. Sensitivity rates vary from less than 20% to greater than 90%, depending on the tumour grade, sensitivity being reduced with well-differentiated tumours.[4] Because of this, it is unlikely to replace cystoscopy for diagnosis.

Renal tract ultrasonography

This is the imaging method of choice for the detection of renal parenchymal disease and urinary tract obstruction. Hydronephrosis will prompt further investigation of the urinary tract distal to the hydronephrosis. Ultrasound is capable of detection and characterisation of renal masses and Doppler facilities allow assessment of the vascularity. However, it is unreliable at detecting upper tract urothelial tumours.

Plain abdominal X-ray

This will detect calcification due to urinary tract calculi, which affect 5% of the population. Calcification may also occur with infection such as tuberculosis or nephrocalcinosis. Nephrocalcinosis is a deposition of calcium salts in the renal parenchyma which may be due to hypercalciuria, renal tubular acidosis or hyperparathyroidism. Renal tumours may cause patchy calcification in 10% of cases.

Cystoscopy

This is recommended in the investigation of haematuria in those over 40 years and anyone with risk factors for bladder malignancy (including frank haematuria). It allows detection of mucosal abnormalities and can be performed reliably with a flexible cystoscope without the need for anaesthesia. This causes less pain and fewer post-procedure problems than the rigid cystoscope. With a general anaesthetic the rigid cystoscope is used to take a biopsy or resect suspicious lesions. Retrograde pyelography can be performed at the same time as cystoscopy if there is doubt about the appearance of the ureters or pelvicalyceal system.

Other investigations

Intravenous urography (IVU) was traditionally the investigation of choice for urinary tract imaging and it remains an important investigation for ureteric calculi or obstruction in patients with haematuria associated with renal colic. It is also indicated if ultrasound is not diagnostic and haematuria persists as it will detect transitional cell carcinoma of the kidney or ureter that ultrasound is likely to miss. However, the sensitivity of IVU is also limited and small renal masses may be missed. Furthermore, IVU cannot distinguish solid from cystic masses and further evaluation with computed tomography (CT) or MRI may be necessary.

CT detects and characterises solid renal masses as well as urinary tract calculi, renal and peri-renal infections and associated complications. The detection rate for renal masses is comparable to that of MRI, and CT is less expensive and more widely available. CT is more sensitive in the detection of renal stones (94–98%) than either IVU (52–59%) or ultrasound scan (19%). CT is therefore the most efficient investigation in differentiating the causes of haematuria and, if used as the investigation of first choice for imaging of the urinary tract, it would reduce the time taken to diagnose the underlying aetiology. However, because of expense and exposure to radiation, it is more commonly used to evaluate abnormalities detected on ultrasound scan or IVU or after negative results from such imaging techniques. MRI is primarily used for tumour staging rather than the initial investigation of haematuria.

Significant proteinuria, renal insufficiency, red cell casts or dysmorphic red blood cells on microscopy should prompt referral to a nephrologist for evaluation of renal parenchymal disease. This may necessitate a percutaneous renal biopsy.

Many urology departments now have one-stop haematuria clinics which aim to achieve a diagnosis at a single outpatient visit. Available investigations include urine cytology, IVU and flexible cystoscopy. Concern has been expressed regarding the potential for over-investigation and unnecessary exposure to ionising radiation.

Prognosis and follow-up

Many women with microscopic haematuria will have no cause found after investigation.[5] Unexplained microscopic haematuria presents a management dilemma. Most centres would discharge such women from further follow-up, although it has been suggested that they should be investigated further with repeat urinalysis, cytology and blood pressure monitoring. More extensive investigations should be prompted by frank haematuria.

References

1. Grossfeld GD, Wolf JS Jr, Litwin MS, Hricak H, Shuler CL, Agerter DC, et al. Asymptomatic microscopic haematuria in adults: Summary of the American Urology Association Best Practice Policy Recommendations. *Am Fam Physician* 2001;63:1145–54.
2. Summerton N, Mann S, Rigby AS, Ashley J, Palmer S, Hetherington JW. Patients with new onset haematuria: assessing the discriminant value of clinical information in relation to urological malignancies. *Br J Gen Pract* 2002;52:284–9.
3. Mariani AJ. *The Evaluation of Adult Hematuria: A Clinical Update.* Houston: American Urological Association; 1998. p. 185–92.
4. Wiener HG, Mian C, Haitel A, Pycha A, Schatzl G, Marberger M. Can urine bound diagnostic tests replace cystoscopy in the management of bladder cancer? *J Urol* 1998;159:1876–80.
5. Bryden AAG, Paul AB, Kyrikides C. Investigation of Haematuria. *Br J Hosp Med* 1995;54:455–8.

KEY POINTS

- All women with haematuria merit investigation with urine micro-scopy, culture, cytology and biochemistry. Renal tract imaging with ultrasound and an abdominal plain radiograph should be performed.

- Frank haematuria or microscopic haematuria in those over 40 years or younger women at high risk should be investigated as above and a cystoscopy should be performed.

- Abnormalities in the urinary tract may require further investigation with IVU and/or CT imaging. These tests will also be required if the above investigations are negative and the woman has frank haematuria or other risk factors for an underlying abnormality.

- Those with significant proteinuria, red cell casts or renal insufficiency should be referred to a nephrologist.

8 Recurrent urinary tract infection

Introduction

Recurrent urinary tract infection is defined as a urinary tract infection that is followed by another infection after resolution of the initial bacteriuria. Often this reinfection is caused by repeated contamination of the urinary tract with perineal flora. Women are much more susceptible to urinary infections than men; at least 20–30% of women will have a urinary tract infection at some time in their life and 25% of these will develop recurrent urinary tract infection.

Bacteria most commonly associated with urinary tract infection are *Escherichia coli* (80%), *Klebsiella* (5%), *Enterobacter* (2%) and *Proteus* (2%). *Staphylococcus saprophyticus* causes 10% of acute cystitis in young women. Anaerobic infections of the urinary tract are rare.

Aetiology

It is unlikely there will be an identifiable underlying abnormality but pathology that should be considered is shown in Table 8.1.

Table 8.1. Pathology that should be considered in the aetiology of recurrent urinary tract infection

Aetiology	Pathology
Anatomical	Bladder or urethral diverticula
	Calculi anywhere within the urinary tract
	Fistulae
	Urethral strictures
	Congenital abnormalities
	Carcinoma
Functional	Incomplete bladder emptying
	Ureteric reflux

Alteration of the vaginal flora may promote the growth of bacteria that are potentially pathogenic to the urinary tract. The glycogen dependent lactobacillus population of the vagina inhibits the growth of *Escherischia coli* and other Gram-negative faecal flora, probably through the production of hydrogen peroxide.[1] After the menopause the glycogen stores in genital tract epithelial cells are depleted and the environment is less supportive of lactobacilli growth. Therefore, there is an increased colonisation of the vagina with *Enterobacter* species and the vaginal pH is higher after the menopause making these women more prone to urinary tract infection.

Some women may be genetically susceptible. It is likely that the adherence and ascent of bacteria through the urinary tract ultimately determine susceptibility to urinary tract infection; the bladder protects itself from pathogen adherence by secreting immunoglobulin A. There may be genetic differences in pathogen receptor availability and binding characteristics at urogenital cells.

Clinical features

Symptoms of lower urinary tract infection include frequency of micturition, urgency, dysuria and suprapubic discomfort. Women with lower urinary tract infection are usually systemically well, but if the infection ascends systemic symptoms such as fever, with or without rigors, malaise, nausea and vomiting occur. Renal angle pain and tenderness are often predominant features of pyelonephritis.

DIAGNOSIS

Urine dipstick analysis for leucocyte esterase activity and bacterial nitrite production is quick and easy. If either test is positive there is 71% sensitivity and 83% specificity for greater than or equal to 1000 colony-forming units (CFU) per millilitre in culture.[2] The diagnosis of urinary tract infection on microscopy remains the gold standard. However, in most laboratories a positive report depends on the presence of greater than or equal to 100 000 CFU/ml; such a high threshold reduces the test's sensitivity. Twenty to fifty percent of symptomatic women have fewer organisms than this; as few as 100 CFU/ml can cause symptoms.[3] Urine must be cultured in the presence of antimicrobials to determine sensitivities.

Investigation

The extent to which recurrent urinary tract infections are investigated is controversial. Tests commonly performed include an estimation of post-void urine residual, cystourethroscopy and imaging of the upper tracts, usually with ultrasound and plain radiography, looking for calculi, evidence of reflux and cortical scarring. However, in the vast majority of women such investigations will prove negative and a degree of clinical discretion is required to prevent the expense and distress caused by over-investigation.

Estimating post-void residual is easy, using a bladder scanner or a catheter, and should be performed on everyone. Further investigation will depend on clinical factors such as the coexistence of haematuria, the severity of symptoms, and the presence of atypical organisms such as *Proteus mirabilis* (which may be indicative of a renal calculus).

IMAGING

Ultrasound scanning is now the primary radiological investigation, having replaced intravenous urography in most centres. The kidneys can be assessed for congenital anomalies such as duplex or horseshoe systems, the cortex can be visualised to investigate scarring from reflux and renal calculi will usually be seen, although visualisation of the mid-portion of the ureter is poor. Ultrasound of the bladder should visualise calculi and diverticula and post-void residuals can be measured.

Intravenous urography will be normal in the majority of women with recurrent urinary tract infection. There is an inherent risk of exposure to radiation and iodine. It is useful in the assessment of the site and severity of ureteric obstruction.

Micturating cystography is occasionally performed if there is recurrent upper urinary tract infection or a suspicion of upper tract damage. It assesses the severity of vesicoureteric reflux, which may require surgical intervention, but it has now been largely superseded by ultrasound scan.

Radionucleide scanning allows calculation of glomerular filtration rates and assessment of the contribution of each kidney to total renal function. It is performed if there is concern regarding renal function, for example if ultrasonography shows evidence of severe cortical scarring from reflux.

Cystoscopy will detect an underlying cause of urinary tract infection such as urethral and bladder diverticula, calculi, foreign bodies, carcinoma or fistulae. Where there are additional symptoms such as pain or haematuria cystoscopy is indicated; in such cases the bladder mucosa needs to be visualised to exclude malignancy and other noninfective inflammatory conditions such as interstitial cystitis. If perfomed using a flexible cystoscope it is a simple and quick outpatient procedure, requiring no anaesthesia.

Treatment

If an underlying cause is found this should be treated. Those who are prone to incomplete bladder emptying should be advised to double void and if necessary be taught to drain their bladder completely at least once daily with clean intermittent self-catheterisation if post-micturition residuals are consistently greater than 100 ml. Urethral dilatation has been commonly used in the past but there is little evidence to support this unless a urethral stricture is present. In the rare cases where severe vesicoureteric reflux is present the kidneys are at risk from scarring and ureteric reimplantation is indicated to protect them.

In the majority of women where investigations are normal conservative treatment includes ensuring an adequate fluid intake (at least 2 litres a day) to try to flush the pathogens away. Women should void frequently and completely as well as voiding before bed and after intercourse. Cranberry juice contains substances such as fructose that inhibit the adherence of a uropathogenic *E. coli* isolate to uroepithelial cells; 300 ml of cranberry juice daily has been proven in a double blind, placebo controlled trial in postmenopausal women to reduce the incidence of bacteriuria with pyuria to 42% of the control group.[4]

Antibiotic treatment is recommended for women with recurrent urinary tract infections. Initially an acute infection should be treated with a short course of an antimicrobial. This can be followed by a prophylactic regimen of low dose antibiotic, which can be taken at night to improve efficacy and compliance or even three times a week. At low doses, the antimicrobial will achieve an adequate concentration in the urine with little effect on the faecal and vaginal flora thereby preventing the development of resistant strains. A single antibiotic can be used and those commonly recommended include trimethoprim, cephalexin, nitrofurantoin and a trimethoprim–sulphamethoxazole combination. They remain effective in the long term despite continued use. Significant resistance does not develop and adverse effects are rare. Some recommend a 3-monthly rotating regimen of differing antimicrobials to minimise any small chance of promoting resistant strains of bacteria. Prophylactic antibiotics reduce the frequency of infections by 95% to less than 0.2 infections per year.[5] Breakthrough infections should be treated with full doses of appropriate antibiotics. Consideration should be given to stopping the prophylactic regimen after six to twelve months to see if the frequency of infections has altered. Some may need to continue daily prophylaxis for life. An alternative to prophylaxis is to allow women to self-medicate. They are provided with 3 days of full dose antibiotic treatment to commence when they suffer the symptoms of acute cystitis. Eighty-five percent of women are able to accurately identify symptoms of a urinary tract infection. The incidence of culture-negative symptomatic episodes, however, is 15%.[6] If the symptoms do not abate promptly the urine should be sent for culture. Patients should be reviewed one week after the infection when another course of antibiotics can be provided for the next episode. Where intercourse is the sole precipitating factor to urinary tract infection women may benefit from a postcoital antibiotic regimen.

Oestrogen should be given to postmenopausal women with recurrent urinary tract infection. By increasing cellular glycogen the oestrogen encourages recolonisation with lactobacilli, thus reducing vaginal pH and inhibiting growth of uropathogens. Postmenopausal women with recurrent urinary tract infections treated with vaginal oestrogen have a marked reduction in symptoms: placebo controlled trials confirm this.[7,8]

References

1. Gupta K, Stapleton AE, Hooton TM, Roberts PL, Fennell CL, Stamm WE. Inverse association of hydrogen peroxide producing lactobacilli and vaginal *Escherichia coli* colonization in women with recurrent urinary tract infections. *J Infect Dis* 1998;178:446–50.
2. Pfaller MA, Koontz FP. Laboratory evaluation of leukocyte esterase and nitrite tests for the detection of bacteruria. *J Clin Microbiol* 1985;21:840.
3. Stamm WE, Counts GW, Running KR Diagnosis of coliform infection in acutely dysuric women. *N Engl J Med* 1982;307:463.
4. Avorn J, Monane M, Gurwitz JH, Glynn RJ, Choodnovskiy I, Lipsitz LA. Reduction of bacteruria and pyuria after ingestion of cranberry juice. *JAMA* 1994;271:751–4.
5. Stapleton A. Prevention of recurrent urinary tract infections in women. *Lancet* 1999;353:7–8.
6. Schaeffer AJ, Stuppy BA. Efficacy and safety of self start therapy in women with recurrent urinary tract infections. *J Urol* 1999;161:207–11.
7. Raz R, Stamm WE. A controlled trial of intravaginal estriol in postmenopausal women with recurrent urinary tract infections. *N Engl J Med* 1993;329:753–6.
8. Cardozo L, Lose G, McLish D, Versi E, de Konig Gans H. A systematic review of estrogens for recurrent urinary tract infections: third report of the Hormones and Urogenital Therapy (HUT) Committee. *Int Urogynecol J Pelvic Floor Dysfunct* 2001;12:15–20.

9 Pregnancy and the renal tract

Many women experience lower urinary tract symptoms during pregnancy and childbirth is commonly cited as the cause for subsequent urinary, colorectal and genital dysfunction. Pregnancy also predisposes to concurrent pathology such as urinary tract infections and hydronephrosis.

Lower urinary tract symptoms

FILLING SYMPTOMS

Between 45% and 90% of pregnant women experience frequency of micturition.[1] This may develop in the first trimester but becomes most noticeable towards the end of pregnancy. It is due in part to the increased production of urine secondary to increased renal plasma flow but in the third trimester the enlarging uterus or presenting part may also cause vesical compression.

Nocturia is often noted for the first time in pregnancy and it is rarely pathological. If defined as at least two nocturnal voids it affects 22–65%[1] of pregnant women. It may be due to increased production of urine and mobilisation of dependent oedema when the legs are elevated during sleep.

Urgency is also common, 60–70% of pregnant women describing the symptom. It has been proposed that high progesterone levels may predispose to detrusor overactivity during pregnancy.[2] However, there is a poor correlation between symptoms and urodynamic findings:[3] detrusor overactivity is confirmed in only one in four women complaining of urge incontinence during pregnancy. Anticholinergic medication is best avoided in pregnancy because of potential adverse effects and toxicity. High doses of oxybutynin have been toxic to the developing fetus in animal studies and manufacturers of tolterodine advise avoidance in pregnancy as no information is available to confirm its safety. Management, therefore, is limited to physiotherapy, caffeine restriction and bladder drill.

URINARY INCONTINENCE

This can present for the first time in pregnancy. Stress urinary incontinence is particularly common, affecting between 32% and 85% of pregnant women. Pressure from the gravid uterus is likely to predispose together with relaxation of smooth musculature and pelvic ligaments secondary to the increase in progesterone and other gestational hormones.

Antenatal stress incontinence frequently resolves after delivery. Pelvic floor exercises are the mainstay of treatment for stress incontinence during pregnancy or immediately after childbirth. Supervised antenatal pelvic floor exercises are effective in reducing postpartum stress incontinence in selected women, including those with increased bladder neck mobility, although efficacy is less apparent when exercises are taught to the general pregnant population.[4,5] Postnatal pelvic floor exercises have been shown to significantly reduce the risk of stress incontinence three months after delivery.[6,7]

Intrapartum events may increase the risk of stress incontinence after delivery. Vaginal delivery, particularly when complicated by prolonged duration of second stage, assisted delivery, third degree perineal tearing and increased birthweight, causes damage to the innervation of the pelvic floor with increased latency of pudendal nerve conduction.[8] There is evidence that vaginal delivery is associated with continence surgery later in life, although this association is confounded by maternal conditions such as body mass index, parity and age at first delivery.[9] Forceps delivery appears to be associated with the development of stress urinary incontinence when compared with vacuum extraction and vaginal delivery.[10–12]

The role of caesarean section is controversial and the published literature is conflicting. There is evidence from a large prospective study of 1169 primiparous women that elective caesarean section may reduce the risk of stress incontinence at six months postpartum.[13] However caesarean section cannot completely prevent urinary incontinence. One study reports that the risk of urinary incontinence is five times higher in women with one or more pregnancies compared with nulligravidae and the risk in women delivered only by caesarean section is still 3.5 times greater than those who have never had a pregnancy.[14] It would therefore appear likely that pregnancy itself as well as delivery causes pelvic floor damage.

VOIDING SYMPTOMS

Approximately one-third of women can experience hesitancy and incomplete bladder emptying. There is often no confirmed voiding disorder on urodynamic testing. Antenatal urinary retention is rare and is most commonly associated with entrapment of a retroverted uterus in the early second trimester. Treatment involves drainage of the bladder, manual reduction of the uterus and possibly a vaginal pessary to maintain anteversion and release the obstruction of the bladder neck.

Epidural anaesthesia, assisted vaginal delivery and caesarean delivery increase the risk of postpartum voiding disorder and retention. All women are however at risk and it is vital that there is careful intrapartum and postpartum bladder surveillance, with prompt catheterisation if retention is suspected. Many women postpartum have decreased bladder sensation: retention may therefore not present with pain. Failing to recognise retention risks overdistension of the bladder with resulting denervation and atony of the detrusor muscle necessitating long-term catheterisation.

COLORECTAL SYMPTOMS

Up to 9% of primiparous women experience anal incontinence three months postpartum and occult sphincter damage is seen ultrasonographically in up to 38% of these women.[15] Assisted delivery and episiotomy predispose.

The risk of postpartum faecal incontinence can be minimised by recognising and repairing the sphincter with appropriate expertise and good analgesia and lighting. It is not known whether an overlapping repair is functionally superior to end-to-end alignment of the anal sphincter;[16] this needs to be subjected to a randomised controlled trial.

HYDRONEPHROSIS

Hydronephrosis is common in pregnancy, secondary to smooth muscle relaxation and pressure on the distal ureter from the gravid uterus. If asymptomatic no action is required. The majority of cases are detected by ultrasound scanning when the woman has presented with pain. Pain relief is usually all that is required. Drainage may be improved by positioning the woman in the knee–chest position. Ureteric stenting performed at cystoscopy or percutaneous nephrostomy using radiological guidance is indicated in symptomatic hydronephrosis that does not respond to conservative management.

URINARY TRACT INFECTIONS

Urinary tract infections are more common in pregnancy, owing in part to progesterone causing smooth muscle relaxation affecting bladder emptying and ureteric drainage. Urinary tract infection is associated with preterm delivery and low-birthweight infants. Maternally, there may be an association with anaemia, hypertensive diseases of pregnancy and diabetes. Because of the morbidity associated with infection, bacteriuria and pyuria are screened for at all antenatal visits using urinalysis dipsticks. Asymptomatic bacteriuria is the presence of 10^5 CFU or more per millilitre. It will develop into acute pyelonephritis in 20–40% if left untreated. Adequate treatment reduces this to 1–2%.

If a urinary tract infection is symptomatic it is termed cystitis. Symptoms may include urgency, frequency, dysuria and frank haematuria. It occurs in 1–3% of pregnant women and it is important to confirm that there is significant bacterial growth on culture.[17]

Pyelonephritis is a systemic illness affecting 1–2% of pregnancies and 70% of these women will have had asymptomatic bacteriuria at the start of their pregnancy. It is associated with fever, rigors, loin pain, nausea and vomiting with bacteriuria or pyuria and leucocyotosis. Women with pyelonephritis should be hospitalised and treated with hydration and intravenous broad spectrum antibiotics. Ultrasound scan should be performed if there is no improvement after 48 hours to exclude stones or obstruction.

All pregnant women who have had a urinary infection should be followed up closely for signs of recurrence. In recurrent cases and cases of pyelonephritis low dose prophylactic broad spectrum antibiotics may be used until delivery. Non-pharmacological prevention of urinary tract infections includes 3- to 4-hourly voiding, pre- and postcoital voiding, increased fluid intake and perineal cleansing.

References

1. Tomezsko JE, Sand P. Pregnancy and intercurrent diseases of the urogenital tract. *Clin Perinatol* 1997;24:343–68.
2. Cardozo L, Cutner A. Lower urinary tract symptoms in pregnancy. *Br J Urol* 1997;80 Suppl 1:14–23.
3. Cutner A, Cardozo L. Assessment of urinary symptoms in early pregnancy. *Br J Obstet Gynaecol* 1991;98:1283–6.
4. Reilly ETC, Freeman RM, Waterfield MR, Steggles P, Pedlar F. Prevention of postpartum stress incontinence in primigravidae with increased bladder neck mobility: a randomised controlled trial of antenatal pelvic floor exercises. *BJOG* 2002;109:68–76.
5. Hughes P, Jackson S, Smith P, Abrams P. Can antenatal pelvic floor exercises prevent postnatal incontinence? *Neurourol Urodyn* 2001;20:447–8.
6. Meyer S, Hohlfeld P, Achtari C, De Grandi P. Pelvic floor education after vaginal delivery. *Obstet Gynecol* 2001;97:673–7.
7. Chiarelli P, Cockburn J. Promoting urinary continence in women after delivery: randomised controlled trial. *BMJ* 2002;324:1241.
8. Snooks SJ, Swash M, Henry MM, Setchell M. Risk factors in childbirth causing damage to the pelvic floor innervation: a precursor of stress incontinence. *Int J Colorectal Dis* 1986;1:20–4.

9. Persson J, Wolner-Hanssen P, Rydhstroem H. Obstetric risk factors for stress urinary incontinence: a population-based study. *Obstet Gynecol* 2000;96:440–45.

10. Arya LA, Jackson ND, Myers DL, Verma A. Risk of new onset urinary incontinence after forceps and vacuum delivery in primiparous women. *Am J Obstet Gynecol* 2001;185:1318–24.

11. Van Kessel K, Reed S, Newton K, Meier A, Lentz G. The second stage of labor and stress urinary incontinence. *Am J Obstet Gynecol* 2001;184;1571–5.

12. MacLennan AH, Taylor AW, Wilson DH, Wilson D. The prevalence of pelvic floor disorders and their relationship to gender, age, parity and mode of delivery. *BJOG* 2000;107:1460–70.

13. Hughes P. Presented at the 26th Annual Meeting of the International Meeting of the International Urogynecology Association, Melbourne, Australia, December 2001.

14. Faundes A, Guarisi T, Pinto-Neto AM. The risk of urinary incontinence of parous women who delivered only by caesarean section. *Int J Gynaecol Obstet* 2001;72:41–6.

15. Chaliha C, Sultan AH, Bland JM, Monga AK, Stanton SL Anal function: effect of pregnancy and delivery. *Am J Obstet Gynecol* 2001;185:427–32.

16. Fitzpatrick M, Behan M, O'Connell PR, O'Herlihy C. A randomised clinical trial comparing primary overlap with approximation repair of third degree obstetric tears. *Am J Obstet Gynecol* 2000;183:1220–4.

17. JFM Santos, RM Ribiero,P Rossi, JM Haddad, HGC Guidi, AM Pacetta, *et al.* Urinary Tract Infections in Pregnant Women. *Int Urogynecol J Pelvic Floor Dysfunct* 2002;13:205–9.

10 Urinary symptoms in elderly women

Lower urinary tract symptoms become increasingly prevalent as women age. Management of symptoms may be challenging: elderly people are less able to tolerate aggressive surgical and pharmaceutical treatments and their symptoms are more likely to be secondary to multiple causes. This chapter will consider the symptoms and pathology that the clinician is likely to encounter in elderly women and how the management differs from the younger population.

Urinary incontinence

Urinary incontinence is a frequent cause of institutionalisation in elderly people. As in younger people, the common causes of urinary incontinence are detrusor overactivity and sphincter weakness. The effects of ageing on the nervous system and lower urinary tract exacerbate the problems encountered in younger people. Furthermore, in up to 35% the pathophysiology of the urinary incontinence may be multifactorial.[1]

As in younger women, it is frequently appropriate to determine the exact cause of incontinence within this group, as it is perfectly feasible to both correct sphincter weakness and treat detrusor overactivity.[2,3] This will often involve urodynamic investigation, the indications for which are outlined in Chapter 4. Cystometry is well tolerated by elderly people although prophylactic antibiotics may be required if they have a predisposition to urinary tract infections. Our threshold for performing a urodynamic assessment is lower in elderly women. This is because empirical treatment based on symptom assessment and a urinary diary alone becomes increasingly unsatisfactory. Elderly people are more likely to have a multitude of co-existing symptoms, and may have multiple pathologies to account for these. They are less likely to tolerate the adverse effects of anticholinergic treatment and drugs risk exacerbating or precipitating urinary retention. It therefore becomes increasingly important to know what the underlying pathophysiology is before treatment.

If detrusor overactivity is confirmed anticholinergic medication can be commenced, but the clinician should be wary of other concurrent medication such as antidepressants that may act synergistically. It is advisable to start with a low dose and gradually titrate the medication until the required benefits are obtained while troublesome adverse effects are kept to a minimum. Detrusor contractility decreases with age and the risk of precipitating urinary retention should be borne in mind. If suspected this can be investigated with free urinary flows and a post-void ultrasound estimate of urinary residual.

Hypermobility of the urethra becomes a less prevalent cause of urinary stress incontinence: the vagina becomes atrophic and vaginal mobility tends to reduce. Therefore, urodynamically proven stress incontinence is more likely to be secondary to intrinsic sphincter deficiency and treatment should be tailored accordingly. Surgery for stress incontinence remains feasible, even in very old women, but general anaesthesia and major abdominal surgery is often best avoided. Treatment with urethral injection therapy (e.g. Macroplastique®, Uroplasty BV, or collagen) or minimally invasive surgical techniques such as the transvaginal tape urethral sling can be performed under either local or regional anaesthesia and are well tolerated. As the detrusor contractility is reduced the risk of postoperative voiding dysfunction is higher in this population. Furthermore, should retention occur elderly women often find self-catheterisation impossible: their eyesight may be failing or they may have reduced manual dexterity. Urethral injection therapy is therefore preferred in frail old women, although the efficacy is lower than a urethral sling, the risk of precipitating urinary retention is also much less.

Urinary frequency and nocturia

The functional capacity of the bladder decreases with age, and bladder filling symptoms such as urgency and frequency become increasingly prevalent.[4] Symptoms require further investigation and a urinary diary is the initial investigation of choice.

Nocturia is particularly prevalent in elderly people. It can be an extremely distressing symptom and is commonly a cause of falls occurring while trying to reach the bathroom. Nocturia in elderly people is frequently secondary to nocturnal polyuria. Diuresis is normally reduced at night, but with nocturnal polyuria more than one-third of the 24-hour urine production occurs at night (see Figure 3.1), perhaps as a consequence of dependent extravascular oedema re-entering the vascular compartment when the lower limbs are elevated in bed. If nocturnal polyuria is evident on the urinary diary, treatment can be implemented, after simple causes such as drinks before bedtime have been excluded. Treatment aims to shift the diuresis to the daytime: loop diuretics 4–6 hours before bed or a small dose of desmopressin before bed have both been shown to be effective.[5] Desmopressin can however result in hyponatraemia, particularly in elderly people, and there is a risk of exacerbating congestive cardiac failure. Consequently it does not currently have a UK licence for this indication. If treatment is commenced it is important to monitor serum electrolytes before and one to three days after commencing treatment, as the hyponatraemia can occur rapidly.

As for younger women, bladder filling symptoms may be secondary to detrusor overactivity, although intravesical pathology such as interstitial cystitis and tumour become increasingly likely and further investigation with urine culture, urine cytology, urodynamics and cystoscopy may be required.

Voiding dysfunction

There is a high incidence of poor detrusor contractility, which can impair voiding even in the absence of outlet obstruction. This may relate to muscle cell degeneration.[6] These factors make elderly women susceptible to urinary retention, which if chronic can be painless and be complicated by overflow urinary incontinence. Bladder outlet obstruction is rare in women, although in elderly women prolapse of the anterior vaginal wall can cause urethral compression and precipitate retention.

Factors that can precipitate urinary retention in elderly women include constipation, drugs (such as alpha-adrenergic agonists or drugs with anticholinergic properties; see below) and bed confinement. These factors probably unmask a previous subclinical voiding dysfunction. Neurological disorders likely to cause voiding dysfunction and retention in elderly women include spinal cord compression secondary to vertebral collapse and spinal cord lesions such as tumours. Strokes impair detrusor contractility initially, but this is commonly later replaced by neurogenic detrusor overactivity, while Parkinson's disease can also cause voiding dysfunction owing to sphincter dyssynergia or poor detrusor contractility.[7] Sensory loss may lead to progressive bladder distension, voiding dysfunction and eventual acontractility and urinary overflow incontinence. Diabetes mellitus is the most common pathology implicated, tabes dorsalis being rare now.

The management of urinary retention becomes increasingly problematic in elderly women. If possible, the treatment of choice, having stopped any implicated medication and rectified reversible factors such as anterior vaginal wall prolapse and concurrent constipation, is self-catheterisation. However, for reasons elucidated above, elderly women frequently are unable to cope with this technique. Drugs to provoke detrusor contractility, such as cholinergics, can be tried but they are frequently ineffective; the main treatment options in these women would include teaching a carer to intermittently catheterise or leaving an indwelling catheter *in situ*. This can be urethral but a long-term suprapubic catheter is likely to be better tolerated as it should not irritate the trigone.

Urinary tract infections

Urinary infections are more common in elderly women, occurring in up to 46% of long-stay geriatric patients over the course of a year.[8] By altering bladder sensation they can cause urinary incontinence, characteristically sensory urge incontinence. Impaired immunological response, voiding dysfunction and urinary stasis, atrophic genital changes, concurrent faecal incontinence and poor fluid intake are some of the factors that predispose to the higher incidence of urinary tract infections in elderly women. There is also a higher likelihood of intravesical pathology and, if of recent onset, recurrent urinary tract infections merit investigation with a flexible cystoscopy. This is well tolerated and usually requires nothing more than a small quantity of anaesthetic lubricating gel. The other investigation of choice is an ultrasound of the urinary tract, looking in particular for incomplete post-micturition bladder emptying.

The majority of women with recurrent urinary infection will however have no identifiable pathology and we would treat with low dose vaginal oestrogen cream, insufficient to cause endometrial proliferation but beneficial to the urothelium. These cells do possess oestrogen receptors and any trophic response may increase urothelial thickness and reduce the likelihood of an ascending bacteriuria. We would also recommend either continuous low dose prophylactic antibiotics or immediate empirical treatment with antimicrobials whenever symptoms recur (see Chapter 8).

Confusional states

Structural brain damage, poor cerebral circulation, metabolic disorders, infections or drug toxicity can cause acute or chronic confusional states, often resulting in the loss of social conditioning with micturition at inappropriate times and in inappropriate places. In addition, neurological pathology is frequently associated with detrusor overactivity and reduced cerebral perfusion may be the cause of 'idiopathic' detrusor overactivity.[9]

Immobility

If the woman suffers with detrusor overactivity, immobility which results in delay getting to the toilet or delay undressing once there can result in urinary incontinence, rather than the frequency and urgency that may be the less troublesome symptoms in the more mobile and dextrous.

Drug therapy

Polypharmacy, or the use of multiple medications concurrently, is common among elderly people. Iatrogenic incontinence is common; up to 60% with incontinence are taking between one and four drugs with potentially adverse lower urinary tract effects.[10] Drugs can adversely affect the lower urinary tract in the following ways:

- **increased urine production**

Diuretic medication, including alcohol, aggravates any lower urinary tract symptoms by increasing the rate of bladder filling.

- **decreased bladder contractility**

Drugs with an anticholinergic action, alpha-adrenergic agonists and calcium blockers all have the potential to decrease bladder contractility. When combined with the poor intrinsic detrusor contractility that can occur in elderly women there is a risk that these preparations can induce urinary retention and subsequent overflow urinary incontinence.

- **increased urethral tone**

Alpha-receptors may be responsible for exerting a tonic sympathetic stimulation on the smooth musculature around the bladder neck and proximal urethra. Phenylpropanolamine has been shown to improve urethral sphincteric insufficiency and there is potential for these drugs to precipitate urinary retention in those with an underlying predisposition.

- **Decreased urethral tone**

Conversely, the use of alpha-blockers can often be correlated with a decrease in urethral profile closure pressures. Beta-adrenergic agonists, particularly those with $beta_2$ characteristics, are able to produce relaxation of slow-twitch skeletal muscle, such as that occurring in the outermost urethral wall. The benzodiazepines also have muscle relaxant effects. The use of all these compounds may therefore reasonably be expected to aggravate urinary stress incontinence.

Conclusions

The approach to urinary incontinence in elderly people differs little from that in younger people. False preconceptions that urinary incontinence in most elderly people is associated with immobility and cerebral disease originate from early reports on geriatric inpatients and it is now accepted that the pathophysiology of incontinence, even in severely disabled elderly people with dementia or severe immobility, does not differ markedly from their peers without such an impairment.[1] Before extensive investigation is embarked on, simple measures should be taken to exclude or rectify constipation, infection, urinary retention and inappropriate medication and to improve mobility and toilet access. Once this has been done evaluation of the lower urinary tract function is recommended; a urodynamic assessment may avoid prolonged medication with inappropriate and poorly tolerated drugs and allow contemplation of surgery. Elderly people should be not denied these benefits on the basis of their age alone.

References

1. Resnick NM, Yalla SV, Laurino E. The pathophysiology of urinary incontinence among institutionalised elderly persons. *N Engl J Med* 1989;320:1–7.
2. Gillon G, Stanton SL. Long-term follow-up of surgery for urinary incontinence in elderly women. *Br J Urol* 1984;56:478–81.
3. Couillard DR, Deckard-Janatpour KA, Stone AR. The vaginal wall sling: a compressive suspension procedure for recurrent incontinence in elderly patients. *Urology* 1994;43:203–8.
4. Swithinbank LV, Donovan JL, du Heaume JC, Rogers CA, James MC, Yang Q, *et al.* Urinary symptoms and incontinence in women: relationships between occurrence, age and perceived impact. *Br J Gen Pract* 1999;49:897–900.
5. Kallas HE, Chintanadilok J, Maruenda J, Donahue JL, Lowenthal DT. Treatment of nocturia in the elderly. *Drugs Aging* 1999;15:429–37.
6. Elbadawi A, Yalla SV, Resnick NM. Structural basis of geriatric voiding dysfunction. III. Detrusor overactivity. *J Urol* 1993;150:1668–80.
7. Malone Lee JG, Wiseman P. Detrusor function in Parkinson's disease. *Neurourol Urodyn* 1991;10:355–6.
8. Brocklehurst JC, Bee P, Jones D, Palmer MK. Bacteriuria in geriatric hospital patients; its correlates and management. *Age Ageing* 1977;6:240–45.
9. Griffiths DJ, McCracken PN, Harrison GM, *et al.* Cerebral aetiology of urinary urge incontinence in elderly people. *Age Ageing* 1994;23:246–50.
10. Gormley EA, Griffiths DJ, McCracken PN, *et al.* Polypharmacy and its effects on urinary incontinence in a geriatric population. *Br J Urol* 1993;71:265–9.

Index